Psychiatry

Mentor

Your Clerkship & Shelf Exam Companion

SECOND
EDITION

Michael R. Privitera, MD, MS
Associate Professor of Psychiatry
Director, Consultation/Liaison Psychiatry Service
Director, Mood and Anxiety Disorder Clinic
Medical Director, Strong Family Therapy Services
University of Rochester Medical Center
Rochester, New York

Jeffrey M. Lyness, MD
Professor of Psychiatry & Associate Chair for
Education
Director, Geriatric Psychiatry Program,
Department of Psychiatry
Director of Curriculum, Offices for Medical
Education
University of Rochester Medical Center
Rochester, New York

F.A. DAVIS COMPANY • Philadelphia

F. A. Davis Company
1915 Arch Street
Philadelphia, PA 19103
www.fadavis.com

Printed in the United States of America

Last digit indicates print number: 10 9 8 7 6 5 4 3 2 1

Acquisitions Editor: Andy McPhee
Developmental Editor: Andrew Pellegrini
Manager of Content Development: George Lang
Art and Design Manager: Carolyn O'Brien

Library of Congress Cataloging-in-Publication Data

Privitera, Michael R.

Psychiatry mentor: clerkship and shelf exam companion / Michael R. Privitera, Jeffrey M. Lyness. — 2nd ed.
p. ; cm.
Rev. ed. of: Psychiatric pearls / Jeffrey M. Lyness. c1997.
Includes bibliographical references and index.
ISBN-13: 978-0-8036-1692-9 (pbk. : alk. paper)
ISBN-10: 0-8036-1692-9 (pbk. : alk. paper)
1. Psychiatry–Handbooks, manuals, etc. I. Lyness, Jeffrey M., 1960- II. Lyness, Jeffrey M., 1960- Psychiatric pearls. III. Title.
[DNLM: 1. Mental Disorders—diagnosis. 2. Mental Disorders—therapy. 3. Psychiatry–methods. WM 141 P961p 2009]
RC456.L96 2009
616.89–dc22   2008030772

To the patients whose lives we endeavor to improve

*To the students, residents, and fellows who have stimulated
our development as teachers*

To our families, for everything

FOREWORD

Psychiatric clerkships are often formidable experiences for medical students, not so much because of the grueling hours and physical exertion, but because psychiatry may seem quite different from other clerkships in medical school. Psychiatric pathology often evokes stronger personal reactions in us than most physical diseases seen, and sometimes encountering the ensuing behaviors that is highly stressful, frightening, or even personally disturbing. Dealing with some patients who may seem weird, crazy, suicidal, or violent can shake up the calmest student's poise.

Issues of personality, emotion, and interpersonal problems may be hard to understand and sometimes strike too close to home. Getting your head around some of the diagnostic concepts in psychiatry may be more difficult, because they often do not lend themselves to neat categories and because there are so few specific laboratory tests to permit "black and white" diagnoses. Trying to understand how these frequently vague clinical syndromes tie in with contemporary neuroscience can be frustrating because the tie-ins are often inexact. Add to that the varying abilities of psychiatric faculty and residents to explain what's going on in plain, simple English. Medical students on their psychiatry rotations may feel as if they are not getting close enough teaching, supervision, or support.

For all these reasons, every student can benefit from a psychiatric mentor. Happily, in this welcome new book, Drs. Privitera and Lyness—two exceptionally experienced and articulate medical student educators in Psychiatry—provide an educational package that addresses the "need to know" facts, concepts, and survival strategies that every clinical clerk will welcome.

Organized around a set of standardized objectives developed by the American Directors of Medical Student Education (ADMSEP), the book starts out with a basic orientation—answers to questions many students would like to ask but don't because they are too embarrassed or because no one is around to answer the questions as they come up. In addition, the introductory section discusses why psychiatry might be important for all students, regardless of the field of medicine they ultimately choose.

The subject matter itself—covering psychiatric assessment, disorders, treatments, and treatment settings—is organized in an easy-to-read fashion, using all the tricks educators have learned to make learning easier for students. There are easy-to-follow algorithms, illustrations, and practical tables.

Mentor Tips are highlighted throughout. These are the wise words you'd hope to hear from instructors, residents, and advisors as you progress through your work. Major learning points are presented telegraphically, so you can read and absorb them quickly. The practice questions provided on the CD-ROM are suitable for self-study or for studying in a group. Because most psychiatric clerkship directors these days place about 25% of the total clerkship grade on shelf exams, these exercises will prove extremely useful.

My guess is that every medical student will find the material in this book extremely useful. I also suspect that psychiatric residents looking over your shoulder who have not had the opportunity to see this book may want to grab it, peruse it, and "borrow" it. So, Mentor Tip: When you're around psychiatric residents, hold on tightly to this book!

Another Mentor Tip: Enjoy your clerkship to the fullest. You're going to be introduced to some of the most profound human experiences you're likely to encounter in your medical career.

Joel Yager, MD

Professor and Vice Chair for Education and Academic Affairs
University of New Mexico School of Medicine
Professor Emeritus, Department of Psychiatry and Biobehavioral Sciences
David Geffen School of Medicine, University of California at Los Angeles

PREFACE

A New Tool for the Clerkship and Shelf Exam

Psychiatric medicine continues to advance, furthering its mission of helping the many people who will suffer from a mental disorder at some time in their lives. In order to give the next generation of clinicians the very best possible study tools, we have created *Psychiatry Mentor,* in which we intend to provide the best preparation possible for the psychiatric clerkship rotation and shelf exam. This book and its accompanying electronic study tools are the next best thing to having a living, breathing mentor by your side 24/7.

Whatever your previous exposure to the field, you no doubt heard many things about psychiatry and psychiatric patients. Some may have been pejorative or led you to worry that you are about to encounter situations that are strange, anxiety-provoking, frightening, or even dangerous. In fact there *are* some important differences between your work in psychiatric settings and that in other medical settings. Learning about these differences is part of the objectives of the rotation. Obtaining good-quality clinical data relies more heavily upon your relationship with the patient as well as from collateral sources of information. However, you will be relieved to discover that most work in this field is highly parallel to work in other medical settings.

As with other rotations, you'll discover that after a week of settling in you will be more clear on your roles and tasks. If you are like most trainees, you'll soon feel comfortable with—even look forward to—coming to work. Such comfort and enjoyment will stem from the inherent fascinating nature of the field (not to mention the brilliance, enthusiasm, and friendliness of your teachers!). The goal of this book, then, is to help you more rapidly reach the point of feeling competent and comfortable. The choice of topics, or more precisely the approach to these topics, is modeled on what students have found important from a variety of sources. Dr. Lyness led the third-year medical student clerkship in psychiatry and is now Director of Medical Student Education in Psychiatry, and Director of Curriculum for the medical school, at the University of Rochester Medical Center. Dr. Privitera has been a clerkship mentor for over 20 years, has run small group seminars for nearly as long, and directed medical student education on the Psychiatry Consultation/Liaison Service at the same institution.

This book is also relevant to other physician trainees newly joining a psychiatry service, whether psychiatry residents or residents from another specialty taking an elective. Many non-physician professional trainees who work in psychiatric settings are likely to find this book useful as well, paralleling the critical roles played by many disciplines in delivering care to the mentally ill.

In this book we consider aspects of the psychiatric rotation itself, including goals, logistics, and approaches to productive and successful clerkship performance. We examine the basics en route to mastering the knowledge base and skills you'll be working on during the rotation. We also discuss the framework within which psychiatric care is rendered, including the settings and the professionals who comprise the relevant staff.

It is our hope that this book will quickly enhance your learning of the fascinating field of psychiatry and more readily allow you to assist the patients in need of your care.

Cross-References to ADMSEP Clerkship Objectives

Standard written objectives for clerkships are a valuable tool—both for teachers, who are responsible for making sure their students learn everything they need to know, and for students, who need an organized summary of what is expected of them. The Association of Directors of Medical Student Education in Psychiatry (ADMSEP) has created such objectives for Psychiatry clerkships (*Academic Psychiatry* 1997; 21:179–204), which are presented at *http://www.admsep.org/appendix.html* Throughout *Psychiatry Mentor,* we have included cross-references to the relevant objectives within that document. Each ADMSEP citation in the *Mentor* text (for example: [II 4-6]) points to a certain objective. This feature shows our readers exactly how each *Mentor* discussion helps to meet the relevant objectives.

A Note About DSM Editions

At the time of writing this book, the edition of the American Psychiatric Association's *Diagnostic and Statistical Manual of Mental Disorders (DSM)* was *DSM-IV-TR*. We expect that the next edition, *DSM-V*, will probably appear within the next several years. We can expect that *DSM-V* will bring important changes to the diagnosis of some kinds of mental disorders. Readers should understand that *DSM-V* will supersede any information herein that, being based on *DSM-IV-TR*, may no longer be definitive, despite having been the very latest information available at the time of this writing.

Michael R. Privitera, MD, MS
Jeffrey M. Lyness, MD
Rochester, New York

ACKNOWLEDGMENTS

MRP would like to thank Dr. Jeffrey Lyness for the opportunity to be part of this education endeavor; Drs. Eric Caine, Glenn Currier, and Steve Lamberti; and Joanne, David, Natalie, and Mark for their encouragement and support on this project.

JML would like to thank Drs. Melissa DelBello, Eric Caine, Yeates Conwell, Laurence Guttmacher, and Mary Lou Meyers for their support and invaluable comments regarding a previous edition of this book, Dr. Privitera for his tireless work on this new and improved edition, and Diane, Colin, Sean, and Trevor for their support, period.

CONTENTS

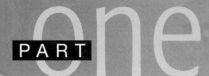

PART one

PSYCHIATRY AS A FIELD OF MEDICINE

CHAPTER 1

INTRODUCTION TO PSYCHIATRY

**Michael R. Privitera, MD, MS, and
Jeffrey M. Lyness, MD**

I. Overview

A. Welcome to your psychiatry experience! Whatever your previous exposure to the field, you have probably heard many things about psychiatry and psychiatric patients. These probably span the range from pejorative to fascinating, frightening to extremely rewarding.
XXIII 9

B. Our purpose is to help you understand your new experience quickly and confidently.

C. You will see parallels to other fields of medicine but rapidly discern and master important differences in psychiatric care.
XXIII 7

II. Definition of Psychiatry

A. Psychiatry: branch of medicine concerned with diagnosis and treatment of persons with mental disorders

1. Applied science and craft

2. Draws on numerous aspects of natural, physical, and social sciences

B. Psychiatrists are physicians who have completed specialty residency training in psychiatry

C. Mental disorder

1. Mental: thoughts, feelings, and actions

2. Disorder: difficulty manifested by subjective distress or observable dysfunction

III. Relevance to Training in Patient Care

A. Why should I learn psychiatry?

1. Interpersonal technical competence

a. All physicians need to develop skills interacting with patients and families.

i. Physician-patient relationship: *primary* tool for gathering data and initiating therapeutic interventions

b. Psychiatry specifically lends itself to learning these skills.

i. Working with and supervision by professionals highly skilled and knowledgeable in this area

ii. Receiving feedback about patient interviews, family meetings, difficult interpersonal interactions (XXIII 2)

iii. Dealing with patients having uncomfortable affects or behaviors: e.g., mute, withdrawn, angry, and so on (XXIII 5-6)

iv. Communicating in difficult situations, (XXIII 6) e.g.:

(1) Cognitive or psychotic impairments

(2) Problems accepting diagnosis

(3) Poor treatment compliance due to limited insight

(4) Problems in ability to understand medical options presented

2. Learning psychopathology

a. All physicians need to understand basics of diagnosis and treatment of psychopathology.

b. Mental disorders are extremely common.

i. These problems found in all fields of medicine

   c. These disorders matter:
      i. Cause functional disability
     ii. Affect individuals, families, others
    iii. Affect outcome of comorbid medical disorders, e.g.,
         increased risk of death from heart disease, cancer
     iv. Can affect compliance with comorbid medical or surgical
         treatments
   d. Psychiatric treatments work.
      i. NIH study: treatments at least as effective as for most
         major physical diseases
   e. Most patients with psychiatric disorders never seek care from
   the "official" mental health system; instead obtain care from
   primary care and other medical specialists.
3. Learning biopsychosocial integration (Figs. 1.1 and 1.2)
   `XXIII 11`

   a. All clinicians routinely encounter and use a wide variety of
   data in planning treatment.
      i. Physical symptoms and exam
     ii. Laboratory results

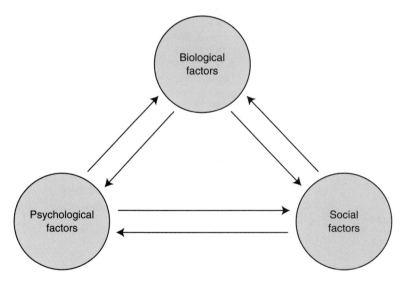

FIGURE 1.1 **Biopsychosocial model.** `XXIII 11`

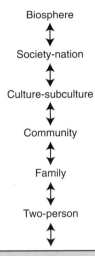

Biosphere
↕
Society-nation
↕
Culture-subculture
↕
Community
↕
Family
↕
Two-person
↕

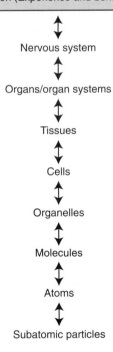

Person (Experience and behavior)
↕
Nervous system
↕
Organs/organ systems
↕
Tissues
↕
Cells
↕
Organelles
↕
Molecules
↕
Atoms
↕
Subatomic particles

FIGURE 1.2 Hierarchy of natural systems in the biopsychosocial model.
XXIII 11

      iii. Behavioral observations of patients and families (including mental status exam)

      iv. Information about social situation and living environment

   b. Psychosocial data are often unstated yet are critical to successful patient care (can be "elephant in the room").

   c. Psychiatry is a good place to learn to integrate three realms of bio-psycho-social issues.

IV. Adjustment to Your Psychiatry Rotation

  A. Understand logistics

    1. Where you need to be and when

    2. Call duties

    3. Role on the team

    4. Responsibilities in patient care

    5. Academic/presentation requirements

    6. Write-up requirements

    7. Learn what is unique to psychiatric patient care

      a. Legal status issues

      b. Confidentiality issues

    8. Preceptor/supervisor—when and how your progress is reviewed

    9. Recommended text(s)

   10. Goals and skills to develop

  B. Usual "phases" of rotation to master

    1. Orientation

      a. Normal to feel like a "fish out of water" first few days to a week

        i. New ways of measuring pathology and clinical changes that are not as concrete as laboratory values or physical findings

      b. Learn how to do psychiatric write-ups

 Focus on observing patients and putting these observations into words (learn the jargon later).

 Focus on observing those more skilled in interviewing. Learn from their experience:

   i. Learn different ways and styles of obtaining clinical data.

   ii. Imagine how you might feel if someone was asking you the questions needed to obtain information.

   iii. Remember sensitivity and respect. XXIII 3

   iv. Some patients may interpret your questioning as implying they are "crazy." Keep to the medical model (and tone)—show that your motive in obtaining information is to help them.

   v. Universalize to set people at ease, e.g.: "When some people get depressed, their mind may play a trick on them. Have you ever had experiences of hearing things or seeing things that were not there?"

 Learn elements of write-ups and doing a mental status exam.

 Multidisciplinary team approach is complex, so try to learn the roles of each discipline.

2. Phenomenology and treatments

  a. Become familiar with official terms (jargon).

  b. Become familiar with array of treatment options (psychotropic medications and psychotherapy).

 DSM criteria become your "friends."

 Apply what you learned from interviews to diagnostic categories.

 Quickest way to get comfortable with therapeutics is to learn psychopharmacology.

   i. After seeing or hearing about how a drug is used, learn how the drug fits into class of drugs and why it is selected.

 Begin to learn when psychotherapy is recommended (in general terms). XXI 4-5

3. Differential diagnosis

    a. You learned phenomenology in different disorders—now work backwards from symptoms (phenomenology) to diagnostic category.

    b. What medical conditions may present with psychiatric syndromes (mimicking primary [idiopathic] psychiatric disorders)?

 DSM has sections on differential diagnosis to assist you.

 Avoid premature closure on a diagnosis.

 Consider pros and cons of a few major diagnostic possibilities.

 Remember to consider possible medical causes of symptoms.

4. Treatment selections

    a. Apply your therapeutic knowledge.

    b. Be able to recommend major treatment options.

        i. When to suggest psychotherapy and for what goals
        XXI 4–5

        ii. What specific medication would you choose and why

    c. Develop some sense of how long a treatment is recommended.

    d. Become familiar with issues that affect treatment.

        i. Personality disorders

        ii. Comorbid medical conditions

        iii. Ongoing stressors

        iv. Other (e.g., support system, cognitive impairments, and so on.)

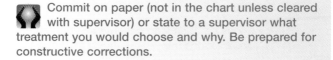 Commit on paper (not in the chart unless cleared with supervisor) or state to a supervisor what treatment you would choose and why. Be prepared for constructive corrections.

Be active on the team in treatment selection decisions.

 Try to learn from as many patients as time permits.

 See the effect of treatment decisions while you are on service.

V. Frequently Used Psychiatric Terms

A. Take some time now to study the terms in **Appendix B: Glossary of Frequently Used Psychiatric Terms.** This group of key terms gets your basic psychiatric vocabulary up to speed. **XXI 3**

VI. Your Evaluation

A. Varies among schools; however, in general:

1. Academic
   a. Fund of psychiatric knowledge
   b. Skills demonstrated
   c. Application of knowledge to clinical reasoning
2. Clinical
   a. Ability to gather and organize data for written and oral presentation
   b. Differential diagnosis and management plan
   c. Procedural skills (for psychiatry, especially mastering mental status exam and interviewing skills for patients and families)
3. Interpersonal
   a. Works well with colleagues and patients
   b. Enthusiasm and energy for subject matter, patient care, and self-education
   c. Professionalism
   d. Receptivity to feedback

 MENTOR TIPS DIGEST

A. Orientation

• Focus on observing patients and putting these observations into words (learn the jargon later).

- Focus on observing those more skilled in interviewing.
- Learn elements of write-ups and doing a mental status exam.
- Multidisciplinary team approach is complex, so try to learn the roles of each discipline.

B. Phenomenology and Treatments

- DSM criteria become your support.
- Apply what you learned from interviews to diagnostic categories.
- Quickest way to get comfortable with therapeutics is to learn psychopharmacology.

C. Differential Diagnosis

- DSM has sections on differential diagnosis to assist you.
- Avoid premature closure on a diagnosis.
- Consider pros and cons of a few major diagnostic possibilities.
- Remember to consider possible medical causes of symptoms.

D. Treatment Selections

- Record (not in the chart unless cleared with supervisor) or state with a supervisor what treatment you would choose and why. Be prepared for constructive corrections.
- Be active on the team in treatment selection decisions.
- Try to learn from as many patients as time permits.
- See the effect of treatment decisions while you are on service.

Chapter Self-Test Questions

Circle the correct answer. After you have responded to the questions, check your answers in Appendix A.

1. Which answer is *incorrect?* Mental disorders:

   a. Affect outcome of comorbid medical disorders.

   b. Are mostly managed by psychiatrists, not primary care and other specialists.

   c. Can affect compliance with comorbid medical or surgical treatments.

   d. Cause functional disability.

2. Difficulty in describing or recognizing one's own emotions (alexithymia) is a common contribution to which type of disorders?

   a. Adjustment disorders

   b. Mood disorders

   c. Schizophrenia

   d. Somatoform disorders

3. The clinician's conscious or unconscious emotional reaction to the patient, determined by the clinician's inner needs, is called:

   a. Countertransference.

   b. Object relations.

   c. Psychosomatic.

   d. Transference.

 See the testbank CD for more self-test questions.

Perspectives on Human Behavior

Michael R. Privitera, MD, MS, and Jeffrey M. Lyness, MD

I. Introduction

A. "Pathogenesis" in psychiatry must be construed more broadly than in traditional pathology and physiology; it should include psychological, and psychosocial, and biological factors.

B. More than one theory may be invoked simultaneously to understand a patient's disorder.
   1. The disorder may be multifactorial.
   2. Different theories may shed important perspectives on essentially same thing.

C. Treatment modalities affect multiple levels of conceptual organization simultaneously.
   1. Antidepressants: ameliorate ideational, affective, and somatic symptoms of depression
   2. Psychosocial treatments: also ameliorate ideational, affective, and somatic symptoms of depression (if mild or moderate level of severity)

D. Theories that provide insight into a disorder do not necessarily lead to effective treatments.
   1. Psychodynamics: gives a rich perspective on obsessive-compulsive disorder, but psychodynamic psychotherapy is ineffective in treating the disorder
   2. Neurobiology: enriches understanding of substance dependence, but psychopharmacology is not a mainstay of treatment for most

II. Genetics (IV 1)
  A. Psychiatric disorders still considered idiopathic
  B. Importance of genetics varies
    1. Largely genetic: pervasive developmental disorder [autism], bipolar disorder
    2. Strongly genetic in some patients and less so in others: major depression
    3. Genetic factors more distant role, or predisposing but not causative: posttraumatic stress disorder, perhaps many personality disorders
  C. Genetic influence is *polygenic* for most disorders: multiple genes in same individual, or different loci in different individuals
  D. In most disorders, genetic influence is *multifactorial:* result of complex interplay between genetic factors and variety of physiological, developmental, psychological, and social events

III. Neurobiology (IV 1-3)
  A. Altered brain function is at least a concomitant of all altered behavior.
  B. Current technology is limited in identifying brain dysfunction.
  C. Whether altered brain function is the cause, contributor, or effect of altered behavior is unknown in most disorders.
    1. Neuroimaging abnormalities may be associated with various disorders.
      a. But this is usually nonspecific
      b. Diagnosis made on clinical grounds
  D. Neurochemistry
    1. Focus on "big three" neurotransmitters [norepinephrine, dopamine, serotonin]
    2. Alterations noted in neurotransmitter activity, turnover, or receptor regulation
    3. Others studied
      a. Acetylcholine: Alzheimer's disease
      b. Gamma-amino butyric acid (GABA): anxiety disorders
  E. Neuroendocrine
    1. Hypothalamic-pituitary-adrenal axis
      a. Studied in mood disorders, stress response, and suicidal behavior
    2. Thyroid function
      a. Mood disorders

3. Female reproductive hormones
F. Psychoneuroendocrinology
  1. Brain and immune system communicate bidirectionally
G. Neuroimaging
  1. Magnetic resonance imaging (MRI) shows more detail than computed tomography (CT)
  2. From crude assessments of brain atrophy or agenesis (total brain volume or ventricular-brain ratio) to specific regions or structures (e.g., dorsolateral prefrontal cortex in schizophrenia or basal ganglia or frontal lobes in depression)
  3. Hopes of determining functional neuroanatomy
    a. Radioisotope labeling
      i. Positron emission tomography (PET)
      ii. Single photon emission computed tomography (SPECT)
    b. Functional MRI
H. Neuropathology
  1. Brain biopsies rarely conducted; usually not illuminating in single cases
  2. Fine-level neuroanatomic abnormalities may be present
    a. Alterations in organization of neuronal architecture in specific cerebral cortical layers in schizophrenia
I. Sleep architecture (by electroencephalogram [EEG] and systemic physiology) altered in:
  1. Mood disorders
  2. Schizophrenia
J. Chronobiology
  1. Seasonal biorhythms
  2. Circadian (daily) biorhythms
K. Neuropsychological testing
  1. Allows examination of cognitive functions that may be tied to particular neuroanatomic regions or pathways

IV. Psychodynamics XXI 1

A. Concepts and theories dominated American psychiatry after World War II and still pervasive in lay images about psychiatry
B. Problems during heyday of psychoanalysis
  1. Other perspectives often excluded
  2. Some practitioners raised expectations too high about ability of psychoanalysis to explain and lead to effective treatment of all mental disorders

C. Psychodynamic perspectives remain fundamental in understanding and working with mentally ill patients.

D. Basic concepts of psychodynamic thought

   1. The unconscious

      a. Much of human mental activity—thoughts, feelings, conflicts, attempts at problem solving—happens outside of conscious awareness.

      b. At least some unconscious activity cannot be brought easily into awareness.

      c. Human behavior that on surface appears irrational or inexplicable may become understandable (although not necessarily reasonable or acceptable) by understanding unconscious processes underlying such behavior.

   2. Defense mechanisms `XXI 3`

      a. Originally, term used for unconscious mental acts that allow individual to mediate ("deal with") unconscious intrapsychic conflicts.

         i. Typical conflict is between wanting something ("id") and simultaneously believing this want is unacceptable ("superego")

      b. Defense mechanisms come into play as a way out of or way to mediate conflict.

      c. The term "defense mechanism" often broadly includes wide range of problem-solving or coping skills, including those that occur consciously and unconsciously. (Table 2.1)

      d. They all work, some better (more fully or more flexibly in a variety of settings) than others.

      e. If person has limited repertoire of defenses or relies on more "primitive" defenses, may not do as well (develop psychiatric symptoms) under certain stressors.

      f. Knowledge of your patient's defense mechanism is useful in managing your treatment alliance and in planning psychotherapeutic treatment.

   3. Transference.

      a. Crucial to understanding patient-physician relationships

      b. When people meet someone new (such as a physician), they bring their sets of expectations, hopes, fears, and emotional reactions to the relationship

TABLE 2.1		
Defense Mechanisms* ADMSEP XXI 3		
Defense	Mechanism	Description
More "primitive" defenses ↑	Denial	Awareness of external reality is kept out of consciousness. May reach delusional proportions (psychotic denial).
	Distortion	Distortion perception or recollection of external reality to meet defensive needs.
	Projection	Unacceptable feelings or wishes are attributed to others. May reach psychotic proportions (e.g., persecutory delusions).
	Projective identification	A more complex defense mechanism that involves a relationship with another person, such as a psychotherapist. Unacceptable feelings or wishes are projected onto the therapist to confirm the projection. (Example: patient with poor self-image projects this on the therapist, with accompanied complaints that the therapist doesn't care about the patient. The patient then acts in such a way to elicit anger or withdrawal by the therapist, thereby "confirming" the projection.
	Splitting	Other people are experienced as either wholly good or bad objects, with associated positive or negative affects. No gray zone exists. This may lead to swings between over idealizing and devaluing others, to creating splits between "good guys" or "bad guys" (e.g., among a multidisciplinary treatment team).
	Acting out	Unacceptable wishes are literally acted upon, but are not experienced consciously.
	Passive-aggressive behavior	Aggression or rage expressed indirectly by inactions such as procrastination or "forgetting" a task.
More flexibly adaptive defenses ↓	Dissociation	A substantial, if time-limited, alteration in one's consciousness, memory, or sense of personal identity.

(continued on page 16)

TABLE 2.1		
Defense Mechanisms* ADMSEP XXI 3 **(continued)**		
Defense	**Mechanism**	**Description**

Left vertical axis label (top): More "primitive" defenses; (bottom): More flexibly adaptive defenses

	Mechanism	Description
	Displacement	Shifting of affects from one object to another, e.g., after a long frustrating day at work (with attendant anger at one's boss), coming home and yelling at one's spouse or kicking the cat.
	Repression	Unconsciously mediated removal of an unacceptable impulse or affect from consciousness.
	Externalization	Related to but broader than projection, involves perceiving one's own attributes and (more often) liabilities in the environment and other persons. Persons with prominent externalizing styles blame circumstances and other people rather than accepting responsibility for their own actions.
	Reaction formation	Consciously experiencing an unacceptable wish or affect as its opposite.
	Intellectualization	Using intellectual processes to minimize or avoid painful affects, impulses, or thoughts. Closely tied to rationalization, in which unacceptable behaviors, thoughts, or feelings are explained away as being reasonable.
	Altruism	Constructively gratifying one's instincts by service to others.
	Anticipation	Reality-based planning for, or worrying about, future inner discomfort.
	Humor	The constructive use of humor to manage difficult thoughts or affects.
	Sublimation	Productively channeling instincts from socially unacceptable to acceptable or desirable ends.
	Suppression	Consciously choosing or planning to postpone attention to a difficult impulse or affect.

*Unconscious, unless otherwise specified.

Adapted from Vaillant GE: *Empirical Studies of Ego Mechanisms of Defense.* American Psychiatric Press, Inc., Washington DC, 1986, pp. 105–117.

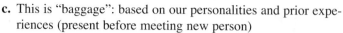

    c. This is "baggage": based on our personalities and prior experiences (present before meeting new person)
      i. Much can be unconscious (not thinking "out loud" about expectations or affects).
      ii. Baggage is real and can profoundly affect the way people view a new person.
    d. In meeting and developing relationship with new physician, complex interplay between preexisting baggage and external reality.
  4. Countertransference
    a. Your own emotional response to a patient colors your interactions.
    b. Is essentially transference of physician toward patient

 Prevent your countertransferences from adversely affecting your interviews and alliance building.

 Develop your skills at altering your interview style or approach in response to specific patient transference patterns.

V. Behavioral Psychology XXI 1

  A. Focus on external, directly observable behaviors
  B. Rooted in learning theory
    1. Specific behaviors can be promoted or reduced by *reinforcers:* responses to the environment that encourage or discourage the behaviors.

 Even natural, helpful responses (e.g., a family's rallying of support in an adolescent girl's suicide attempt) can serve as a positive reinforcer to undesired behavior (suicidal behavior). Thus, clinical goal is to help this patient meet her needs without using suicidal acts.

  C. Behavioral techniques used with a variety of disorders and symptoms
    1. All have in common: encouraging (reinforcing) desired behaviors and discouraging (extinguishing) dysfunctional or dangerous behaviors.

2. Cognitive psychology (XXI 1)
   a. Studies the way people think
   b. In psychiatric disorders, describes characteristic ways people think while suffering from particular emotional states such as depression or panic attacks
      i. Emotional states stem from problematic thinking
      ii. Dysfunctional patterns of thoughts occur automatically and lead to affective symptoms and other components of the disorders
      iii. *Cognitive distortions* may affect how one views oneself, external environment, or future (Table 2.2).
      iv. In cognitive therapy, patients learn to identify their dysfunctional thoughts and replace them with more functional, less distorted thoughts

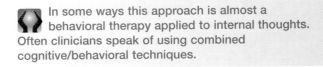

In some ways this approach is almost a behavioral therapy applied to internal thoughts. Often clinicians speak of using combined cognitive/behavioral techniques.

VI. Group Psychology (XXI 1)
   A. Theories that focus on understanding human behavior manifested in groups
   B. Groups manifest their own properties, affected by:
      1. Properties of individuals in group
      2. Group size
      3. Goals or tasks
      4. Leadership
   C. Theories of small group dynamics underlie approaches to group psychotherapy
   D. Important also in nonclinical work, such as psychological assessment of organizations (e.g., corporations)

VII. Family Systems (XXI 1)
   A. Families are complex systems that have their own characteristic patterns of interaction, both within family and in relation to rest of world (including physician).
   B. Behavior within a family takes on a complexity that must be understood at the level of the family.

TABLE 2.2	Examples of Cognitive Distortions
Distortion	**Essential Characteristics**
Dichotomous thinking (all-or–nothing thinking)	Perceiving things as either/or, black/white, good/bad, and so forth
Minimization or maximization (catastrophizing)	Selectively prioritizing the importance of certain facts, such as dwelling on one critical comment made by a coworker while ignoring his or her many praising comments
Overgeneralization	Basing broad, sweeping beliefs on few or single incidents
Arbitrary inference (jumping to conclusions)	Coming to a belief or conclusion without direct evidence
Personalization	Taking events personally without evidence for such a connection
Selective abstraction (mental filter)	Dwelling on one small part of a more complex, larger situation
Disqualifying the positive	Rejecting positive experiences by insisting that they "do not count", despite contradictions by everyday experiences
Emotional reasoning	Assuming that negative emotions reflect the way things really are
Should statements	Motivating yourself (if guilt) or others (if anger, resentment, frustration) with "should"s and "shouldn't"s
Labeling and mislabeling	An extreme form of overgeneralization; attaching a negative label to yourself or others

Adapted from Burns DD: *Feeling Good.* Avon Books, 1999.

1. Understand the individuals, but also in the context of their role in the family
2. Family interaction becomes more than a sum of individuals
C. A patient presenting with psychiatric symptoms cannot be fully understood without appreciating his or her family history and current state.

    D. Meetings with family may be essential for data gathering as well as assistance to achieve successful psychotherapeutic ends.

VIII. Developmental Perspectives 🔟
    A. No single, catch-all developmental theory
    B. Human development occurs in several areas across life span
        1. Physiological
        2. Psychological
        3. Interpersonal factors
    C. May be several theories or perspectives of single domains, such as personality
    D. Two broad perspectives worth considering as you formulate each patient
        1. Where is your patient now in his or her developmental course, and how successfully (or not) has he or she been in adapting to demands of current developmental needs and challenges?.
        2. Developmental perspective may offer insights into current behavioral patterns as influenced by earlier life experiences.

> It is important not to oversimplify, e.g., blaming everything about a patient's difficulties on "bad parenting." Yet, it would be a reasonable postulation that, for example, repeated childhood abandonment by foster caregivers has contributed to a 20-year-old's current poor sense of self and tendency toward depressive symptoms and self-destructive acts.

  IX. Other Perspectives
    A. *Cultural:* recognize profound influence of culture on psychological and interpersonal processes and on expression of, and response to, psychopathology, as well as on attitudes toward psychiatric and general medical care
    B. *Interpersonal:* focus upon patient's interaction with others; as a form of psychotherapy (Interpersonal Psychotherapy, IPT) can be very effective in treating, for example, major depression
    C. *Couples:* draws upon family and interpersonal theories, with focus upon a two-person system (dyad)

D. *Ethics:* perspectives in all of medicine, in psychiatry major focus related to autonomy and consent

E. *Forensic psychiatry* ⟨ XIX 5–8 ⟩: includes legal aspects in usual psychiatric care (informed consent, confidentiality, involuntary commitment to treatment) and those interfacing with criminal justice system (relationship of mental disorder to criminal actions, competency to stand trial, etc.)

F. *Community psychiatry* ⟨ XIX 1–4, 9–10 ⟩: focus upon populations, psychopathology from epidemiological perspective, consideration of health services delivery by studying, modifying or designing psychiatric systems of care for large numbers of mentally ill persons

 MENTOR TIPS DIGEST

- Prevent your countertransferences from adversely affecting your interviews and alliance building.
- Develop your skills at altering your interview style or approach in response to specific patient transference patterns.
- Even natural, helpful responses (e.g., a family's rallying of support in an adolescent girl's suicide attempt) can serve as a positive reinforcer to undesired behavior (suicidal behavior). Thus, clinical goal is to help this patient meet her needs without using suicidal acts.
- In some ways patients learning to identify their dysfunctional thoughts and replace them with more functional, less distorted thoughts is almost a behavioral therapy applied to internal thoughts and often clinicians speak of using cognitive/behavioral techniques.
- It is important not to oversimplify. Yet, it would be a reasonable educated speculation to postulate, for example, that childhood repeated abandonment by foster care givers has contributed to a 20-year-old's current poor sense of self, and tendency toward depressive symptoms and self-destructive acts.

Resources

Burns DD: Feeling Good. Avon Books, 1999.

Vaillant GE: Empirical Studies of Ego Mechanisms of Defense. American Psychiatric Press, Inc., Washington DC, 1986, pp 105–117.

Chapter Self-Test Questions

Circle the correct answer. After you have responded to the questions, check your answers in Appendix A.

1. More than one theory of human behavior may be invoked simultaneously to understand a patient's disorder because:

   a. A patient's disorder may be multifactorial.

   b. Different theories have equal effectiveness for each disorder's treatment.

   c. Theories that help us understand a disorder necessarily lead to effective treatments.

   d. Treatment modalities affect one level of conceptual organization at a time.

2. Of the following, the psychiatric disorder with the strongest genetic component is:

   a. Bipolar disorder.

   b. Major depression.

   c. Personality disorder.

   d. Post-traumatic stress disorder.

3. Neuroendocrine studies that are thought to be important in psychiatric disorders include all of the following *except:*

   a. Aldosterone regulation.

   b. Female reproductive hormones.

   c. Hypothalamic-pituitary-adrenal axis.

   d. Thyroid function.

4. All of the following are true about neuroimaging studies in psychiatry *except:*

    a. Crude assessments of brain atrophy or agenesis have been studied.

    b. Hopes of determining functional neuroanatomy from radioisotope labeling.

    c. MRI shows less detail over CT.

    d. Specific regions or structures have been studied.

5. Which of the following is not one of the three major neurotransmitters best studied in psychiatric disorders.

    a. Dopamine

    b. Glycine

    c. Norepinephrine

    d. Serotonin

See the testbank CD for more self-test questions.

PART two

PSYCHIATRIC WORKUP

HISTORY AND PHYSICAL EXAMINATION

**Michael R. Privitera, MD, MS, and
Jeffrey M. Lyness, MD**

I. Introduction

   A. Psychiatric workup: similar in broad outline and in many details to general medical workup you have been doing.

   B. Important points of refinement (although applicable in other settings) will be highlighted in psychiatry.

   C. Become accustomed to and skilled at gathering and organizing psychological and psychosocial data with the same rigor and detail you employ with gathering data on physical symptoms, laboratory values, and other "objective" data.

   D. Psychiatric syndromes can be ascertained with same degree of reliability as most general medical data.

II. Elements of History and Physical (Table 3.1) 11-12
A. Identifying data
1. *Who:* demographic description of patient
2. *How:* method of referral
   a. Self-referred
   b. Sent by general medical provider
   c. Sent by another mental health provider
   d. Psychiatry inpatients: mention patient's legal status in your write-up, such as voluntary or involuntary
3. *Why:* briefly but descriptively: *your* sense of most important or most prominent part of patient's presentation
B. Chief complaint
1. *Patient's* words on what he or she sees as most prominent reason for presenting for care
2. Use direct quotes or paraphrases whenever possible

> In psychiatry, comparison between identifying data (ID) and chief complaint (CC) can be illuminating; e.g., "ID: This is a 26-year-old single white male admitted from the emergency department on an involuntary status with paranoid delusions after being mental hygiene arrested. CC: 'There's nothing wrong with me, you should be locking up my neighbors after what they did to me!'"

C. History of present illness (HPI)
1. Describes what patient is presenting with, but complexities exist for clinician (as in all fields of medicine) as to the following questions
   a. Do I have full story?
   b. When did presentation actually begin?
   c. How do I best organize data to describe it?
2. Do I have full story?
   a. Sources of information 12
      i. Patient
      ii. Relatives or friends
      iii. Treaters or other staff involved in patient's care
      iv. Old records
   b. Make clear at beginning of your workup what your data sources are, and estimate their reliability and completeness

TABLE 3.1

Psychiatric Workup [ADMSEP I 1,4,5]

Element	Description
Identifying data	Age, race, gender, marital status, referred by whom for what?
Chief complaint	Presenting symptoms, organized syndromically if possible, and their chronology/context
Medications	List all; specify outpatient vs. current inpatient medications if the patient is an inpatient
Past psychiatric history	Substance-use history; prior psychiatric syndromes, treatments (include psychotropic medication history and psychotherapy)
Past medical and surgical history	The usual
Family history	Psychiatric and medical family history; genogram; family relationship patterns
Developmental/ social history	Role performances throughout life course; current living and social circumstances
Review of systems (ROS)	The basic medical ROS, plus any relevant psychiatric ROS not already covered
Physical exam	The usual, but pay careful attention to the neurological exam

Mental status exam	A significant part of what you're here to learn. Components include:
	• General appearance and behavior
	• Quality of relationship with interviewer
	• Psychomotor activity
	• Speech
	• Mood and affect
	• Thought content
	• Thought process
	• Perceptual disturbances
	• Cognitive functions
	  • Level of consciousness
	  • Orientation
	  • Attention
	  • Memory
	  • Language
	  • Fund of knowledge
	  • Visuospatial skills

(continued on page 28)

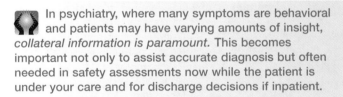

TABLE 3.1	
Psychiatric Workup ADMSEP I 1,4,5 (continued)	
Element	**Description**
	• Calculations • Frontal executive functions • Abstraction • Judgment and insight
Laboratory values	All current (and any recent and relevant) blood work, neuroimaging studies, etc.
Diagnostic impressions	The Five Axes of DSM
Formulation	How do you understand the nature and potential etiology of the patient's presenting problems? (can include relevant differential diagnosis in this section)
Problem list and plan	All relevant psychiatric and medical problems and all relevant biological, psychological, and social interventions

In psychiatry, where many symptoms are behavioral and patients may have varying amounts of insight, *collateral information is paramount.* This becomes important not only to assist accurate diagnosis but often needed in safety assessments now while the patient is under your care and for discharge decisions if inpatient.

    c. At some point (based on urgency to get your write-up into the chart), make decision to stop and write up what you have now, knowing it may later be supplemented or supplanted by what you eventually learn
        i. Consider putting in "plan" section what you intend to do to complete database information-gathering II 6-8

Accept this limitation calmly and humbly, realizing it goes with the territory.

3. When did presentation actually begin?

  a. Easier for new recent-onset illness, not so easy for patients with prior episodes, symptoms, or treatment encounters

  b. No one right way to do HPI; do what seems most clinically sensible

> As in other fields of medicine, there may be ambiguity to what is considered onset of symptoms; e.g., a patient with schizophrenia may have had an admission last year, began using cocaine the last 6 days, and began escalating psychosis and suicidal focus the last 6 hours before coming to the emergency department. Do your best to figure what is most related to the current state, but can reference previously diagnosed with schizophrenia in HPI, with more detail about this previous diagnosis (dx) in "Past Psychiatric History" section. Most likely in this case, it would be best to consider the episode onset around the time of the recent cocaine use—was this use independent of worsening psychotic symptoms, or as a result of worsening symptoms?

4. How do I best organize data?

  a. Most common organizer used by neophytes is *chronology*

   i. Advantage: simplicity; an overarching conception of patient's illness is not necessary—just report the order events occurred

   ii. Disadvantage: reader needs to pull data together from different parts of chronology to develop a conception of patient's illness

  b. Better and tighter HPIs use *syndromic approach*

   i. Analogy: like arguing a legal brief

   ii. Strands of history in HPI (pertinent positives and negatives) should be filtered and organized to lead inexorably to "closing argument"—formulation and differential diagnosis

  c. Begin HPI with terse description of patient's presenting symptoms, clustered together as much as possible

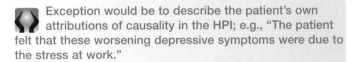

For example, "Ms. Xanadu developed depressive symptoms including persistently depressed mood with daily crying spells, feelings of worthlessness, early morning awakening by 2 hours, and weight loss of 17 pounds. . . . She also noted increasing 'nervousness,' which was present continuously but with some variation in degree. Along with this anxiety, she had dry mouth, tremulousness, and nausea."

d. As part of symptom descriptions, include relevant "dimensions" of symptoms

e. Use terse examples to help flesh out your descriptions

For example, after mentioning that a patient had persecutory delusions, convey the content of these delusions: "He felt that his neighbors had tried to poison his food."

f. Describe context within which patient experiences symptoms

For example, "Anxiety was first noticed after a disruptive argument with spouse."

g. Describe general stressors or significant events that have taken place during time of presentation of symptoms

For example, "Patient has many difficult-to-meet deadlines at work and learned of the death of a cousin."

h. Do not make premature attributions of causality in relation to stressors—save such causal speculation for the formulation

Exception would be to describe the patient's own attributions of causality in the HPI; e.g., "The patient felt that these worsening depressive symptoms were due to the stress at work."

i. Include pertinent negatives

> For example, for a patient with severe depressive symptoms, state "no suicidal ideation or diurnal variation." If patient has delusions, include "no hallucinations or gross thought process disruption." Differential diagnosis drives whether a "negative" is truly pertinent (in *syndromic approach* described earlier).

   j. Chronological approach can now be used to describe what patient tried to do for his or her symptoms, in temporal order; description should conclude clearly explicating how patient came to present to you today

> For example, "The daughter called the police after her father threatened her with a knife; he was brought to the emergency department under mental hygiene arrest."

D. Medications `I 12`
   1. Full list of all medications (psychotropic and nonpsychotropic) with dosage schedules if known
   2. Indicate drug compliance
   3. Describe any recent medication or dose changes and when they occurred
   4. Inpatients: list outpatient medications prior to coming into hospital as well as current inpatient medications

> Making effort to distinguish outpatient versus inpatient medications helps to more quickly discern possible reasons for new inpatient symptoms; for example: anxiety and nightmares if selective serotonin reuptake inhibitors (SSRIs) were not continued (SSRI discontinuation syndrome), or delirium and seizures if benzodiazepines were not continued (benzodiazepine withdrawal)

   5. Ask about over-the-counter medications, vitamins, supplements, herbals, and topical agents
E. Past psychiatric history
   1. Substance use history: you may have been taught to include in social history, but this demeans direct relevance to physical and mental disorders

a. Substance used
b. Doses or amounts
c. Chronology, including frequency and patterns of use
d. Review of pertinent positives and negatives regarding abuse and dependence
   i. Alcoholic blackouts
   ii. Withdrawal symptoms
   iii. Attempts to cut down or quit
e. Describe any formal outpatient or inpatient substance-abuse treatments
f. Under social history, you might include psychosocial circumstances of substance use, e.g., drinking after work, on weekends with spouse, etc

2. Other past psychiatric history
a. Need to ask in several ways to get a complete picture

   `III 1–10`

   i. Have you ever seen a psychiatrist or other mental health professional? ("counselor" or "therapist" may trigger a patient's recall)
   ii. Have you ever been counseled by your primary care physician for emotional troubles?
   iii. Have you ever been given a "nerve pill" or "sleeping pill" by a physician?
   iv. Have you ever been hospitalized for emotional or psychiatric reasons?
   v. Have you ever tried to harm or kill yourself in the past? (may be surprising how many people tell you "yes" after denying all prior queries about emotional troubles or treatment)
   vi. "Yes" answers should lead to a series of questions designed to elicit specifics
      (1) What diagnoses were given?
      (2) What specific symptoms were present?
      (3) What treatments were used (including details of medication trials as doses, duration, adverse effects)?
      (4) Response to treatments and subsequent course—did they return to baseline?
   vii. In addition to formal history of psychiatric treatment, ask about past syndromes that may have been untreated or long forgotten

(1) "Was there ever a time in your life where you felt sad or blue much of the time for a couple weeks on end?" "What about a period when your mood was unusually happy, giddy, or on top of the world?"

(2) For females who have had children, it may be useful to ask about postpartum depressive symptoms or other postpartum symptoms of relevance.

3. Time lines, sometimes called *life-charting*, are a useful way to rapidly and visually summarize course and progression of illness, when there have been previous episodes (Fig. 3.1).

F. Past medical and surgical history

1. Because you have spent the rest of your training on this section, we do not dwell on the details; do not skimp on this section just because it is a "psych patient" ▮ I 10-11 ▮

   a. Medical illnesses are highly comorbid with psychiatric disorders and are often directly relevant (physiologically or otherwise) to psychiatric presentation

G. Family history

1. As done in other settings (e.g., genogram, usual disorders may be conveyed), but ask specifically about psychiatric disorders

2. As mentioned in past history, may have to do some creative (i.e., clear and specific) questioning

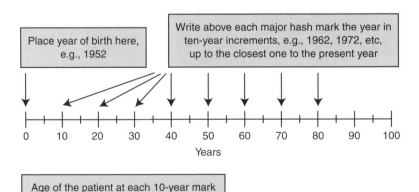

Place year of birth here, e.g., 1952

Write above each major hash mark the year in ten-year increments, e.g., 1962, 1972, etc, up to the closest one to the present year

0   10   20   30   40   50   60   70   80   90   100

Years

Age of the patient at each 10-year mark

FIGURE 3.1 Patient life chart. Mark on the chart when past episode(s) of illness occurred and any brief associated useful detail such as hospitalizations, suicide attempts, first medication treatments, etc.

    a. Formal contacts with mental health system
    b. Untreated, suspected syndromes
    c. Hospitalizations (or in "old days," institutionalizations)
    d. Suicide attempts and completions
    e. Alcohol and other substance abuse problems
  3. If elicit a positive family history, attempt to determine details as diagnoses, treatments (including specific medications) if known
  4. Can include relationships among family members; relevant aspects of cultural, socioeconomic, or religious background; prominent or enduring patterns of (mis)communication; areas of alliance or discord—especially between patient and others
H. Developmental/social history
  1. Developmental history
    a. Fundamental importance to a full psychodynamic understanding of patient and may yield clues to etiology or clinical phenomenology of current condition

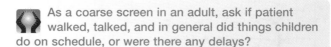

Clinical setting, patient condition, and time available dictate practicality of obtaining developmental history.

    b. Full developmental history
      i. Any complications in utero
        (1) During pregnancy with, or delivery of, the patient
      ii. Developmental milestones (as learned in Human Development and Pediatrics)
        (1) Motor
        (2) Cognitive
        (3) Social

As a coarse screen in an adult, ask if patient walked, talked, and in general did things children do on schedule, or were there any delays?

      iii. School years
        (1) Completed grades as scheduled
        (2) Special or remedial education
        (3) Specific grades achieved
        (4) Social roles: network of friends; how relate to parents, siblings, others in household

      iv. Adolescence
         (1) Same questions as above
         (2) Dating history
         (3) Sexual history
      v. Early adulthood—domains of concern are social and occupational
         (1) Spouse or other love/sexual relationships
         (2) Friends
         (3) Community, religious, sports, or hobby-related organizations
         (4) Other avocational group affiliations
         (5) A careful job history, noting patterns of difficulty with maintaining employment, and try to specify what led to any troubles: interpersonal conflict; inability to work effectively
      vi. Continue these tasks as you move through adulthood
         (1) How patient performed developmental tasks
         (2) Reaction to expected or unexpected stressful events: raising children, illnesses, financial or other job losses, children leaving household, job promotions or lack thereof, retirement
  2. Social history
    a. Current living environment
      i. Physical location and layout
      ii. Who lives there
      iii. Help available
    b. Occupation and how well it is going
      i. Job performance
      ii. Interpersonal relationships at work
    c. Religious or other subcultural or community affiliations
    d. Current social environment
      i. Important people in their life
      ii. How much contact with these persons
      iii. Qualitative nature of these relationships
      iv. Socioeconomic conditions
      v. Functional abilities (if not already clear from HPI and physical history)
      vi. Daily routine of patient
I. ROS

1. Usual medical ROS

 Do not sell "psych patients" short on thoroughly evaluating physical symptoms.

2. Use this section to check that you asked about all relevant current and past psychiatric symptoms as well as physical symptoms

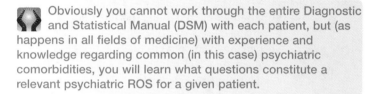 Obviously you cannot work through the entire Diagnostic and Statistical Manual (DSM) with each patient, but (as happens in all fields of medicine) with experience and knowledge regarding common (in this case) psychiatric comorbidities, you will learn what questions constitute a relevant psychiatric ROS for a given patient.

J. Physical exam
1. Give due diligence to your physical exam because of the high comorbidity of general medical and mental disorders (I 10-11)
2. Also pay close attention to a careful screening neurological exam
3. With evidence from the medical history, general physical, or cognitive exam suggesting likelihood of neurological disease, do a more extensive neurological exam
4. In severe mental illness, especially note nonlateralizing neurological findings, often associated with primary as well as secondary psychiatric disorders, and side effects of psychotropic medications (I 10-12)
   a. Adventitious movements (dyskinesia, tremors)
   b. Subtle dysarthrias
   c. Gait abnormalities

 MENTOR TIPS DIGEST

- In psychiatry, comparison between identifying data (ID) and chief complaint (CC) can be illuminating; e.g., "ID: This is a 26-year-old single white male admitted from the emergency department on an involuntary status with paranoid psychosis after being mental hygiene arrested. CC: 'There's nothing wrong with me, you should be locking up my neighbors after what they did to me!'"

- In psychiatry, where many symptoms are behavioral and patient may have varying amounts of insight, *collateral information is paramount.* This becomes important not only to assist accurate diagnosis, but often needed in safety assessments now while the patient is under your care and for discharge decisions if inpatient.
- Accept calmly and humbly the limitation of beginning your write-up of HPI with only the information you have, realizing it goes with the territory.
- Just as in other fields of medicine, there may be ambiguity as to what is considered onset of symptoms; e.g., a patient with schizophrenia may have had an admission last year, began using cocaine the last 6 days, and began escalating psychosis and suicidal focus the last 6 hours before coming to the emergency department. Do your best to figure what is most related to the current state, but you can reference previously diagnosed as schizophrenic in HPI, with more detail about this previous dx in the "Past Psychiatric History" section. Most likely in this case, it would be best to consider the episode onset around the time of the recent cocaine use—was this use independent of worsening symptoms, or as a result of worsening symptoms?
- Example of beginning HPI with terse description of patient's presenting symptoms, clustered together as much as possible: "Ms Xanadu developed depressive symptoms including persistently depressed mood with daily crying spells, feelings of worthlessness, early morning awakening by 2 hours, and weight loss of 17 pounds. . . . She also noted increasing 'nervousness,' which was present continuously but with some variation in degree. Along with this anxiety, she had dry mouth, tremulousness, and nausea."
- Use terse examples to help flesh out your descriptions; e.g., after mentioning that a patient had persecutory delusions, convey the content of these delusions: "he felt that his neighbors had tried to poison his food."

- Example of describing the context within which the patient experiences symptoms: "Anxiety was first noticed after a disruptive argument with spouse."
- Example of describing general stressors or significant events that have taken place during time of presentation of symptoms: "Patient has many difficult-to-meet deadlines at work, and learned of the death of a cousin."
- Exception to not making premature attributions of causality in the HPI would be if the patient attributes such causality, such as "The patient felt that these worsening depressive symptoms were due to the stress at work."
- Example of including pertinent negative if severe depressive symptoms would be "no suicidal ideation or diurnal variation." If the patient has delusions, include "not hallucinations or gross thought process disruption." Differential dx drives whether a "negative" is truly pertinent (in *syndromic approach* described earlier).
- Example of using chronological approach when describing what patient tried to do for his or her symptoms, then ending up how patient came to present to you today, would be: "The daughter called the police after her father threatened her with a knife; he was brought to the emergency department under mental hygiene arrest."
- Making effort to distinguish outpatient versus inpatient medications helps to more quickly discern possible reasons for new inpatient symptoms. For example: anxiety and nightmares if SSRIs were not continued (SSRI discontinuation syndrome), or delirium and seizures if benzodiazepines were not continued (benzodiazepine withdrawal).
- Clinical setting, patient condition, and time available dictate practicality of obtaining developmental history.
- As a coarse screen of developmental history in an adult, ask if patient walked, talked, and in general did things children do on schedule, or were there any delays?
- Do not sell "psych patients" short on the competency or your evaluation of physical symptoms.

- Obviously you cannot work through the entire Diagnostic and Statistical Manual (DSM) with each patient, but (as happens in all fields of medicine) with experience and knowledge regarding common (in this case) psychiatric comorbidities, you will learn what questions constitute a relevant psychiatric ROS for a given patient.

Chapter Self-Test Questions

Circle the correct answer. After you have responded to the questions, check your answers in Appendix A.

1. Which of the following elements is not put in the Identifying Data section of the psychiatric write-up?

   a. Demographic description of the patient

   b. Method of referral

   c. Patient's words on most prominent reason for presentation

   d. Your sense of the most important part of the patient's presentation

2. Which of the following is not a significant reason for obtaining collateral information about the patient?

   a. Many psychiatric symptoms are behavioral, and therefore another source can clarify or support presentation of symptoms.

   b. Others have a right to know the symptoms of the patient.

   c. Patients may have varying degrees of insight and may not be aware of their symptoms.

   d. Safety decisions such as discharge of a patient may be assisted by input from someone who knows the patient baseline for comparison.

3. Which of the following is not an advantage of organizing the HPI in the syndromic method?

   a. It is more tightly organized.

   b. Data are pulled together to give a conception of the illness.

   c. Pertinent positives and negatives are filtered and organized to lead to the formulation and differential diagnosis.

   d. You do not have to have an overarching conception of the patient's illness, you just have to describe events in order.

4. What is necessary to be able to classify data as pertinent positives or pertinent negatives?

   a. An overarching conception of the patient's illness

   b. Knowing the order in which the symptoms occurred

   c. Memorization of DSM criteria

   d. Patient's words on what he or she sees as most prominent reason for presenting for care

5. When describing the History of the Present Illness, in which of the following situations is it easiest to describe as to when the illness began?

   a. Patients with a previously diagnosed axis one disorder plus a new factor that may mimic the disorder such as illicit drug use

   b. Patients with chronic symptoms but a new stressor

   c. Recent onset illness

   d. Those with one previous episode compared with more than one

See the testbank CD for more self-test questions.

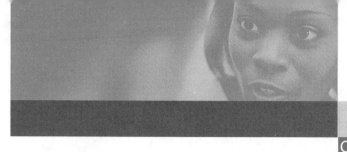

CHAPTER

MENTAL STATUS EXAMINATION

**Michael R. Privitera, MD, MS, and
Jeffrey M. Lyness, MD**

I. Overview

A. Mastering mental status exam (MSE) is major goal of psychiatry
rotation ❨14-5❩
B. MSE is analogous to physical exam (PE)
  1. Terse language
  2. Organized way of observing and reporting findings from time of
contact with patient
  3. Should merely describe data

 Save interpretations of your data for assessment/
formulation sections.

C. MSE should describe only data observable during interview
with patient

 If patient was noted or reported to have hallucinated
several hours before interview but not during interview,
hallucinations should be mentioned in the history of present
illness (HPI) or review of symptoms (ROS), whereas in the MSE,
note "no hallucinations at this time."

D. Many textbooks suggest writing MSE in paragraph form
  1. Suitable for experienced MSE writers

2. For trainees, more useful to write MSE as list with headings suggested as follows: (analogous to PE: "HEENT, Lungs, Cardiac, etc.")
   a. General Appearance and Behavior
   b. Quality of Relationship to Interviewer
   c. Psychomotor Activity
   d. Speech
   e. Mood and Affect
   f. Thought Content
   g. Thought Process
   h. Perceptual Disturbances
   i. Cognitive Functions
   j. Judgment and Insight

> Using list headings in the MSE will help you get comfortable quickly with the crucial skills of breaking down your behavioral observations into components.

E. MSE covers *wide range* of mental experiences and manifestations, of which cognition is only one part
   1. Too often, term "mental status" incorrectly used synonymously with "cognitive status" e.g., "mental status changes"
   2. Trained observers can describe most of MSE after *any* patient interview
F. Part of goal of developing MSE skills is to use relevant technical jargon properly (with all advantages of terseness and precision that jargon is supposed to provide)
   1. Avoid redundancy

> In general medicine, e.g., you would not say "the patient had rales, with a crunchy kind of sound audible through a stethoscope." You would simply say "the patient had rales." Similarly, in psychiatry, you would not say "the patient's thought processes were tangential; he was unable to stick to one subject and tended to drift from one topic to another." You would simply say "the patient was tangential."

   2. Adjectival specifiers are useful; e.g., "mild tangentiality"

II. Components of MSE

A. General appearance and behavior

1. This and next section "set the stage" for rest of MSE
2. Things to consider and possibly comment on include:
   a. Level of hygiene and grooming
   b. Choice of clothing—more than aesthetics—is it appropriate to environment, weather, situation, etc.? (e.g., T-shirt and shorts in snowy weather, sunglasses while inside, garish clashing colors, perfectly pressed gray pinstripe suit, etc.)
   c. Where is patient seen? (e.g., in bed, while pacing in hall)
   d. Are there unusual motor activities or mannerisms?
   e. Does patient appear his or her age?

B. Quality of relationship to interviewer

1. Comment tersely on manner in which patient related to you
   a. Eye contact: "none," "fair," "occasional," "good," or "normal"; "excessive," "intense," or "unwavering"
   b. Tone of relationship: "warm," "neutral," "reserved," "hostile," or "angry"; "guarded," "suspicious," "flirtatious," or "seductive"; "withdrawn" or "totally unengaged"
      i. These qualities may vary, so describe them as such: "He was initially hostile, but engaged progressively and well by the interview's end."

C. Psychomotor activity

1. Technically, might include all motor behavior observed during interview
2. In practice, includes all such activity beyond what was already described in motor section of neurological exam
3. In abbreviated reports (without neurological exam), this is the place to describe evident tremulousness, tics, dyskinesias, akathisia, or choreiform movements

 If psychomotor movements dominate overall appearance of patient, mention in "General Appearance" section as well.

   a. Unusual motor activity
      i. Posturing movements
      ii. Waxy flexibility (sustained posturing combined with potential for passive manipulation of position)

    b. Motor hypoactivity (psychomotor retardation)
      i. Slowness of verbal responses (increased speech latency)
      ii. Slowing of movements or decreased initiation of movements
    c. Hyperactivity (usually psychomotor agitation): give specifics

> There is a lot of difference between hand wringing (or leg rocking or foot tapping) and pacing with fists clenched. It is useful to *describe* the agitation. Do not merely say "agitated" because that gives no sense of the quality and severity of the agitation. It is possible to have both agitation and retardation at the same time. See Chapter 9 on "Psychobiological Parameters and Clinical Presentations" for more discussion.

D. Speech
  1. Encompasses physical production of verbal output

> Remember the distinction between "speech" and "language." Speech is the *physical production* of oral communication. Language refers to the *cognitive (intellectual) function* of generating and expressing thoughts in verbal/communicable form, which may be expressed by oral speech, sign language, writing, or other means.

    a. Dysphonia (trouble with production of vocal "wind"; e.g., hoarseness) or hypophonia (decreased vocal wind)
    b. Dysarthria (trouble with articulation)
    c. Volume
    d. Amount (if increased, may be referred to as *logorrhea*)
    e. Speed
    f. Modulation and inflection (*dysprosody* is term for loss of normal speech melody)
    g. Spontaneous versus responsive only
    h. Latency (see Psychomotor Activity)
    i. Pressured speech (a sense of force or pressure behind words, even beyond volume, amount, or speed, that makes it hard to interrupt)
E. Mood and affect
  1. Terms to describe patient's emotional state

2. Principle distinctions that are described
   a. Mood:affect::climate:weather
      i. Mood is overall prevailing emotional state during
         interview
      ii. Affect is the variability of emotions during course of
          interview
   b. Mood includes subjective elements expressed by patient
   c. Affect focuses more on objective elements, e.g., what is
      observed of patient.

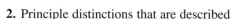 Often, mood is determined by asking patient about
it (e.g., "How would you describe your mood, your
spirits?") Quote patient when possible, but feel free to offer
own assessment if different from verbatim response.

3. Words to describe mood: neutral, sad/depressed/down,
   happy, euphoric, expansive (meaning maximum euphoric),
   anxious/tense/nervous/worried, etc.; irritable (easily angered),
   angry
4. Affect domains
   a. Intensity: how much emotion is expressed or excluded? If
      severely reduced: "flat" or "blunted"
   b. Range: affect stuck in one position or varies? If varies,
      describe how: "from neutral to tearfulness to mild anger"
   c. Appropriateness: is patient's affect congruous with thought
      content?
   d. Lability: does affect shift from one emotion to another with
      abnormally rapid, all-or-none quality?

In conceptualizing lability, think of turning on a
water spigot from off to full pressure in a flash. In
neurological or neuropsychiatric settings, if especially
inappropriate to content is often described as "emotional
incontinence," "pseudobulbar affect," or "inappropriate
emotional expression."

   e. Reactivity: does affect change appropriately with shifts in
      thought content, or truly unchanging? Sometimes described as
      an attribute of mood.

F. Thought content

  1. Briefly highlight prominent themes, especially if relate to presenting problems; e.g., nihilistic or guilty themes (depressed patient), grandiose themes (manic patient), etc.

  2. Presence or absence of "abnormal" thought content

    a. Delusions (firmly held false beliefs that are not culturally bound)

    b. Suicidal or homicidal ideation

      i. Ask about gradient of self-destructive thoughts (from thoughts of just hurting self physically as self-injurious behavior to thoughts of wanting to die or kill themselves).

> In assessing suicidal ideation you might ask "Have you had thoughts that life is not worth living?" Follow this with: "Have you thought about wanting to die or wanting to take your own life?" In assessing homicidal ideation: "Have you ever had thoughts about harming someone else?"

      ii. In MSE document descriptions of:

        (A) Ideation.

        (2) Plans. (Does patient have method in mind?)

        (3) Intent. (Is patient at point of thinking he/she may actually do it?)

      iii. Put previous suicide attempts or homicide attempts in HPI or Past History as appropriate

    c. Obsessions

    d. Overvalued ideas (unshakable convictions not false enough to count as delusions)

    e. Poverty of content (paucity of ideas or topics, as seen in delirium, dementia, depression, or negative symptoms of schizophrenia) `16`

> Give examples or descriptions of any abnormal thought content; e.g., "persecutory delusions are present, with beliefs that his telephone is being tapped by the FBI."

G. Thought process

  1. Concerned with flow of patient's ideas and how well they connect with one another.

2. Terms for normal thought process: logical, goal-directed, well-organized
3. Terms to describe thought process "derailments," i.e., disruptions in goal-directed process
   a. *Tangentiality:* literally, going off on a tangent; that is, starting on one topic and, in linear fashion, straying off topic until patient (and listener) is far from original topic

    Mild forms of tangentiality may be found in normal persons, but severe forms are a form of psychosis.

   b. *Circumstantiality:* literally, talking around the topic at hand, often getting back to the topic but not speaking directly about main issue

    Circumstantiality may range in severity from normal to psychotic.

   c. *Thought blocking:* patient's train of thought suddenly comes to a halt, and so does his or her verbal output
   d. *Loosening of associations:* topics shift from one subject to another in an unrelated or oblique manner, leaving the listener with no idea of how the patient got from "point A to point C"; when severe, can be incomprehensible speech
   e. *Flight of ideas:* classically seen in manic syndromes; patients move rapidly from one topic to another, usually across several topics in a rapid sequence 16

   Compare flight of ideas (comprehensible relationship between topics when shifting, but rapid sequence) with loosening of associations (incomprehensible relationship between topics when shifting, at any speed). Both can exist at the same time.

   f. *Word salad:* words and phrases mixed together that lack logical coherence or comprehensible meaning; classically seen in schizophrenic patients, although can be part of any severe psychosis 16

g. *Ruminative thinking:* tendency to dwell on same theme; in severe forms occurs despite interviewer's attempt to shift attention

 The term "perseveration" is often misused to refer to ruminative thinking; it really refers to a cognitive problem (shifting attention). See the cognitive section on attention below.

h. Other descriptors of thought process disturbance (fascinating but less common)
   i. *Echolalia:* repetitious echoing of words or syllables uttered by another
   ii. *Clang associations:* uttering words that rhyme, alliterate, or otherwise associate by sound rather than meaning (e.g., "I fell and hurt my right *arm*, so I had to *arm* myself, as the *Arm*y's *arm*amentarium is large.", "I tried to knock clock fox pox.")
   iii. *Punning:* linking phrases only by use of homonyms, not by their sense (e.g., "*Auntie* Rita must be a gambler as she likes to *ante* up.")

H. Perceptual disturbances
   1. Abnormalities of sensory perception
      a. *Hallucinations:* sensory perceptions wholly without external basis
         i. Auditory (most common)
         ii. Visual
         iii. Olfactory
         iv. Tactile
         v. Gustatory
      b. Be sure to ask patient directly if any unusual sensory experiences
         i. "Do you ever hear things that other people don't hear?"
      c. Some patients deny having hallucinations, but "appear to be responding to internal stimuli"; therefore describe what you observe

There is an enormous stigma about mental illness or particularly about being "crazy" that is deeply rooted in our culture (think how you might feel if someone asked whether you heard voices). Therefore, ask questions about hallucinations sensitively; it is usually best if you have first established some relationship with the patient through other questions that establish a medical setting context. The reason for this suggestion is twofold: your patient will be less embarrassed when answering in the positive, and you are more likely to obtain positive answers if they truly exist.

For simplicity, delusions are often combined in MSE with hallucinations (e.g., "patient did not have any delusions or hallucinations"). However, remember distinction between them: *delusions:* thought content disturbance; *hallucinations:* sensory disturbance.

    d. *Illusions:* gross distortions of actual sensory input (e.g., the sound from walking on dry leaves being perceived as voices, or a clock on the wall being perceived as someone's face staring at the patient)
I. Cognitive functions
  1. Overview
    a. Cognition: complex, multidimensional range of intellectual functions encompassing all the various modes of knowing and reasoning

Try to distinguish between true cognitive impairments and those of motivation. If patient says, "I don't know," does that answer really reflect, "I don't want to try"?

    b. Cognitive assessment range of tests
      i. Observation during interview
        (1) Important complement to more formal bedside testing
        (2) Can be done based on any patient interview
          (A) Level of consciousness
          (B) Attentiveness
          (C) Orientation to surroundings (note if not "formally tested")
          (D) Recall of recent or remote events (note if not "formally tested")

(E) Language
(F) Visuospatial skills (e.g., asking ambulatory patients to find their rooms or other destination, or asking nonambulatory patients to describe how they would get to their destination)

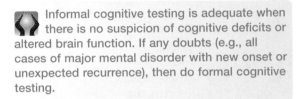 Informal cognitive testing is adequate when there is no suspicion of cognitive deficits or altered brain function. If any doubts (e.g., all cases of major mental disorder with new onset or unexpected recurrence), then do formal cognitive testing.

ii. More formal bedside testing
  (1) Mini Mental State Examination (MMSE) (Table 4.1)
    (A) Well-validated in certain populations
    (B) Less usefulness in acutely ill psychiatric patients
    (C) Drawbacks
      (i) Emphasizes total score (e.g., 23/30), but realms of deficits are clinically more important
      (ii) Some realms (e.g., frontal lobe function) poorly covered by MMSE
      (iii) Patient loses points for wrong answers, no matter how close (yet close versus far off matters clinically)

TABLE 4.1	
MMSE Total Score Interpretation	
Patient Demographics	**Interpretation Clues**
If <70 years old and ≥ high school education:	30 → Normal, not ill, probably not demented
	≤25 → behavioral syndrome may be secondary to cognitive impairment
	≤22 → probably demented (if arousal and concentration are normal)
If non-ill and little education	22–26 → common range
If active primary Axis I syndrome	27–29 → common range
If ≥+++++80 years old	25 → average

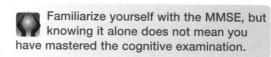

Familiarize yourself with the MMSE, but knowing it alone does not mean you have mastered the cognitive examination.

    (2) Conceptualizing brain function by location can assist with clinical correlation (Fig. 4.1)

    (3) Other testing (see below)

  iii. Neuropsychological testing

    (1) Extensive, specific, well-standardized tasks using pen, paper, blocks, and other prepared materials

    (2) Requires doctoral-level psychologist (i.e., Ph.D. or Psy.D.) with special training to interpret

2. Level of Consciousness (LOC)

  a. Most common cognitive component documented in patient charts

  b. Exists on a continuum

  c. Normal: alert

  d. Range: Hyperalert/hypervigilant, alert, lethargic, obtunded, stupor, coma

Lethargy is defined as lowered LOC but able to be aroused to alert, although perhaps only briefly (e.g., "he was lethargic, arousable to voice but only for a few seconds at a time"). Coma is defined as unarousable unresponsiveness to external stimuli. Stupor and obtundation are between lethargy and coma, although the boundaries between them may be less distinct.

3. Orientation

  a. Second most common cognitive component documented in patient charts

  b. Genuinely useful quick screen of cognition

  c. A multidetermined function, relies on level of consciousness, language skills, memory, attention to environmental cues, etc.

  d. "Oriented × 3" = person, place, and time

    i. Person (specify what tested, and response if incorrect): self, interviewer's name, role of other people?

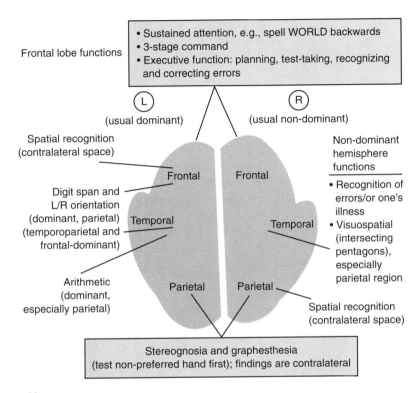

Frontal lobe functions
- Sustained attention, e.g., spell WORLD backwards
- 3-stage command
- Executive function: planning, test-taking, recognizing and correcting errors

(L) (usual dominant) (R) (usual non-dominant)

Spatial recognition (contralateral space)

Digit span and L/R orientation (dominant, parietal) (temporoparietal and frontal-dominant)

Arithmetic (dominant, especially parietal)

Frontal   Frontal

Temporal   Temporal

Parietal   Parietal

Non-dominant hemisphere functions
- Recognition of errors/or one's illness
- Visuospatial (intersecting pentagons), especially parietal region

Spatial recognition (contralateral space)

Stereognosia and graphesthesia (test non-preferred hand first); findings are contralateral

Memory:

Function	Subserved by
New learning	Parahippocampal cortex Cerebellar neocortex (when motor responses involved)
Storage	Hippocampus, amygdala, cerebellum, cerebral neocortices
Recall	Anterior mesial-temporal areas

FIGURE 4.1 Brain function by location.

Orientation to interviewer is very heavily dependent on how long and how well the patient has known the interviewer. It is often more useful to limit "orientation to person" to mean orientation to self.

ii. Place (specify what tested and response): state, city, county, hospital name, floor, part of the hospital (e.g., emergency room, medical floor, psychiatric floor)
iii. Time (specify what tested and response): day of the week, date, month, season, and year
  e. If patient has difficulty: try multiple-choice cues to see if patient can pull out correct answers (see tips on cueing under "Memory" below)
4. Attention
  a. Attention is indistinguishably tied to concentration (although subjective report of concentration may be different from actual performance on formal tests of attention)
  b. Impaired in two ways
    i. Difficulty sustaining attention
      (1) Formal Tests
        (A) "serial 7s"—although this task also depends heavily on calculation skills as well as on education level (e.g., subtracting 7s from 100: 93, 86, 81,78,71; patient got only two correct out of five)
        (B) "WORLD backwards" (e.g., DLRWO; patient got three out of five correct)
        (C) "A" random letter test—steady, slow stream of random letters; patient raises hand when hears "A"
    ii. Difficulty shifting attention from one task to next
      (1) Verbal perseveration (e.g., to the question "What is the month?" the patient responds "August." To the next question "What year is it?" the patient answers "August." To the third question "What floor are you on?" the patient answers "August."
      (2) Visuomotor perseveration (see testing for perseveration under Frontal Executive Functions later)
5. Memory
  a. Complex realm of functions
  b. Subtypes: immediate/short-term/long-term or verbal vs. non-verbal memory
  c. Testing short-term memory (see Fig. 4.1)
    i. Registration: repeat three objects
    ii. Recall after 5 minutes

(1) *Free recall:* spontaneously remembered without need for cues
(2) If free recall fails, try *categorical cue:* if apple was object: "It was a kind of a fruit"
(3) After categorical cue fails, try *word list cueing:* multiple choices in list, "Was it a pear, apple, or banana?"

 Your documentation after testing short-term memory might read "patient registered 3 objects easily, recalled 1/3 at 5 minutes, 2/3 with categorical and 3/3 with word list cues."

Distinguish between problems retrieving a memory and storing it; if cueing helps, "deficit was more retrieval than storage."

  d. Testing long-term memory
    i. Includes asking about recent and remote events
      (1) Recall of HPI
      (2) Major news events or themes of the day: widely known topic or something this patient would be expected to know based on education and sociocultural background
      (3) More remote memory
        (A) Over-learned details, e.g., birth date, wedding date, and names of siblings or children.
        (B) Major news events of past years
          (i) Age ≥75 years: Pearl Harbor
          (ii) Age ≥55 years: President Kennedy's assassination
          (iii) Age ≥35 years: Space shuttle Challenger explosion
          (iv) Age ≥15 years: 9/11/2001 terrorist attacks on U.S. targets

6. Language
  a. Patient's vocabulary: appropriate to education?
  b. Word-finding difficulties or other problems with fluency evident in conversation?
  c. Paraphasic errors

   i. Complete word substitution: semantic paraphasia (e.g., "I
      wrote down the message with my *car*"—instead of "pen")
   ii. Syllable substitution: phonemic paraphasia (e.g., "I wrote
      down the message with my *ten*"—instead of *p*en)
   iii. Replacement with word that does not exist: neologistic
      paraphasia (e.g., "I wrote down the message with my
      shrip"—the word *shrip* does not exist)
  d. Dysnomic dysphasia: ask to name objects
   i. Commonly: "pen" or "watch"
   ii. Subtle naming: e.g., parts of watch
   iii. Cannot name but tells what it does: circumlocutory error
  e. Repetition dysphasia: repeat short syllable phrases as "no ifs
    ands or buts," or "Methodist Episcopal"
  f. Verbal fluency: in one minute name as many words as possible
    that begin with "d" or things that can be found in grocery store.
  g. Comprehension: follow commands, answer questions appropri-
    ately in a way that demonstrates understanding of the question
  h. Writing: useful for patients with difficulties with speech or
    spoken verbal fluency
7. Fund of knowledge
  a. Very affected by intelligence, education, and cultural back-
    ground
  b. Current or past events
  c. Some standardized questions exist: e.g., "Where does rain
    come from?"
8. Visuospatial skills
  a. Variety of pencil-and-paper tasks
   i. Common: copy figures (square, intersecting pentagons)
   ii. Draw a clock, and add "put hands at 10:10"; increases the
     difficulty; therefore, more sensitive to deficits
  b. Place actual attempts in chart, instead of just describing
  c. Ambulatory patients: do they find their room or other nearby
    destination
  d. Nonambulatory patients: describe how they would get to such
    a destination
9. Calculations
  a. Arithmetic skills (while affected by education and native
    intelligence) may be impaired specifically in cognitive deficit
    disorders.

b. Ask to perform one-step operations: "How much is 15 plus 17?" "What is 4 times 6?"

c. Make problems simpler, if necessary.

d. Alternatively ask about making monetary change: "If you had a dollar and bought a newspaper for 25 cents, how much change would you receive?"

10. Frontal executive functions (FEFs)

  a. Least tangible and hardest to describe of cognitive functions, yet affected by many brain-disease processes and crucial to daily functioning

  b. Involved in organizing, prioritizing, sequencing, and executing a variety of mental and physical actions

  c. Patients with diseases affecting frontal lobe structure and function may demonstrate such difficulties

  d. MMSE includes three-step command for FEF

  e. Involves shifting attention (overlapping with concept of perseveration)

  f. Bedside tests

   i. Testing for motor perseveration at bedside (Fig. 4.2)

 Errors repeating the same diagram component: graphomotor perseveration.

Ask patient to copy this diagram:

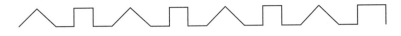

Example of motor perseveration:

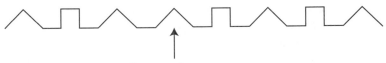

Perseverative error

FIGURE 4.2 Testing for motor perseveration.

ii. Perform three motions with one hand sequentially on either a table or knee, repeat as rapidly as possible
(1) Pound (fist)
(2) Cutting motion (edge of hand)
(3) Patting motion (with palm prone)

 FEF three-motion test: observe for slowness, perseverative errors (e.g., fist twice before edge), sequence errors (e.g., fist, palm, edge). Errors not accounted for by motor weakness may be ascribed to frontal lobe dysfunction on contralateral side. **16**

11. Abstraction
   a. Substantial portion of the adult population, by dint of intelligence, education, or cultural background, functions at fairly concrete level
   b. Proverb interpretation, often cited in texts, may be heavily influenced by cultural background and whether heard before
   c. Better to ask about similarities
      i. Start with example, then give test: "a car and boat are both transportation; how are an apple and banana similar?"

Interpretation of similarity between apple and banana abstraction

(1) "Both fruits": abstract response
(2) "Both have skin": concrete response
(3) "Both red": wrong response
(4) "Both offspring of the earth and part of Nature's grand plan": hyperabstract (suggests possible expansive mood)
   d. Ask about differences
      i. Example: "Which of the following does not belong with the others: a boy, a door, or a man?"
J. Judgment and insight
   1. Judgment
      a. In general way, ability to plan and act wisely and in accord with established cultural norms
      b. Assessment

     i. Ask what the patient would do in certain circumstances: "What would you do if you smelled smoke in a movie theatre?"

    ii. Acutely ill patients: more useful to assess based on recent actions leading to clinical presentation, e.g., brought by police wandering in subzero temperatures without warm clothing

2. Insight

  a. Accuracy and depth of understanding of a situation (clinical context: into own illness or troubles)

  b. How well patient's understanding of illness jibes with yours, or what was the patient told by previous physicians?

    i. Does patient accept that anything may be wrong or externalize all blame on others?

  c. How does patient respond when you explain (in appropriate language) your assessment of condition or need for treatment?

 MENTOR TIPS DIGEST

- Save the interpretations of your data for the assessment/formulation sections.
- If the patient was noted or reported to have hallucinated several hours before the interview but not during the interview, hallucinations should be mentioned in the HPI or ROS, whereas in the MSE, note "no hallucinations at this time."
- Using list headings in the MSE will help you get comfortable quickly with the crucial skills of breaking down your behavioral observations into components.
- In general medicine, e.g., you would not say "the patient had rales, with a crunchy kind of sound audible through a stethoscope." You would simply say "the patient had rales." Similarly, in psychiatry, you would not say "the patient's thought processes were tangential; he was unable to stick to one subject and tended to drift from one topic to another." You would simply say "the patient was tangential."
- If psychomotor movements dominate the overall appearance of the patient, mention in "General Appearance" section as well.

- There is a lot of difference between hand wringing (or leg rocking or foot tapping) and pacing with fists clenched. It is useful to *describe* the agitation. Do not say "agitated" because that gives no sense of the quality and severity of the agitation. It is possible to have both agitation and retardation at the same time. See Chapter 9 on "Psychobiological Parameters and Clinical Presentations" for more discussion.
- Remember the distinction between "speech" and "language." Speech is the *act* of verbal communication. Language refers to *any means of communicating* characteristic of a person, group, profession, or technical device.
- Often mood is determined by asking patient about it (e.g., "how would you describe your mood, your spirits?") Quote patient when possible, but feel free to offer own assessment if different from verbatim response.
- In conceptualizing lability, think of turning on a water spigot from off to full pressure in a flash. In neurological or neuropsychiatric settings if especially inappropriate to content is often described as "emotional incontinence," "pseudobulbar affect," or "inappropriate emotional expression."
- In assessing suicidal ideation you might ask, "Have you had thoughts that life is not worth living?" Follow this with: "Have you thought about wanting to die or wanting to take your own life?" In assessing homicidal ideation: "Have you ever had thoughts about harming someone else?"
- Give examples or descriptions of any abnormal thought content; e.g., "Persecutory delusions are present, with beliefs that his telephone is being tapped by the FBI."
- Mild forms of tangentiality may be found in normal persons, but severe forms indicate psychosis.
- Circumstantiality may range in severity from normal to psychotic.
- The term "perseveration" is often misused to refer to ruminative thinking; it really refers to a cognitive problem (shifting attention).

- Compare Flight of Ideas (comprehensible relationship between topics when shifting, but rapid sequence) to Loosening of Associations (incomprehensible relationship between topics when shifting, at any speed). Both can co-exist at the same time.
- There is an enormous stigma about mental illness or particularly about being "crazy" that is deeply rooted in our culture (think how you might feel if someone asked whether you heard voices). Therefore, ask questions about hallucinations sensitively; it is usually best if you have first established some relationship with the patient through other questions that establish a medical setting context. The reason for this suggestion is twofold: your patient will be less embarrassed when answering in the positive, and you are more likely to obtain positive answers if they truly exist.
- For simplicity, delusions are often combined in MSE with hallucinations (e.g., "patient did not have any delusions or hallucinations"). However, remember distinction between them: *Delusions:* thought content disturbance; *Hallucinations:* sensory disturbance
- Try to distinguish between true cognitive impairments and those of motivation. If patient says, "I don't know," does that answer really reflect, "I don't want to try"?
- Informal cognitive testing is adequate when there is no suspicion of cognitive deficits or altered brain function. If any doubts (e.g., all cases of major mental disorder with new onset or unexpected recurrence), then do formal cognitive testing.
- Familiarize yourself with the MMSE, but knowing it alone does not mean you have mastered the cognitive examination.
- Lethargy is defined as lowered LOC but able to be aroused to alert although perhaps only briefly (e.g., "he was lethargic, arousable to voice but only for a few seconds at a time"). Coma is defined as unarousable, unresponsiveness to external stimuli. Stupor and obtundation are between lethargy and coma, although their boundaries may be less distinct.

* Orientation to interviewer is very heavily dependent on how long and how well the patient has known the interviewer. It is often more useful to limit "orientation to person" to mean orientation to self.
* Your documentation after testing short-term memory might read "patient registered 3 objects easily, recalled 1/3 at 5 minutes, 2/3 with categorical and 3/3 with word list cues."
* Distinguishing between problems retrieving a memory and storing it can be achieved. Cueing can aid retrieving a memory, but not if storing the memory is a problem.
* Errors repeating the same diagram component: graphomotor perseveration
* FEF three-motion test: observe for slowness, perseverative errors (e.g., fist twice before edge), sequence errors (e.g., fist, palm, edge). Errors not accounted for by motor weakness may be ascribed to frontal lobe dysfunction on contralateral side.
* Interpretation of similarity between apple and banana: may be abstract, concrete, wrong, or hyperabstract

Resources

Folstein MF, Folstein SE, and McHugh PR: Mini-Mental State, a practical method for grading cognitive state of patients for the clinician. Journal of Psychiatric Research 12:189–198, 1975.

Taylor MA: The Fundamentals of Clinical Neuropsychiatry. Oxford Press, 1999, pp. 80–104.

Chapter Self-Test Questions

Circle the correct answer. After you have responded to the questions, check your answers in Appendix A.

1. The Mental Status Examination (MSE) is analogous to the physical examination in that it:

   a. Compares previous findings with present ones.

   b. Interprets findings.

c. Is an organized way of observing and reporting findings from time of contact with patient.

d. Records superfluous findings.

2. Most of the MSE can be described by a trained observer after:

   a. Any patient interview.

   b. Consultation with a neuropsychologist.

   c. Formal cognitive testing.

   d. Neuroimaging.

   e. Only a very lengthy patient interview.

3. In the Quality of Relationship to Interviewer section of the MSE, which of the following is included?

   a. Eye contact

   b. Level of hygiene and grooming

   c. Unusual motor activities

   d. Where the patient is seen

4. An example of *adventitious* motor activity is:

   a. Decreased initiation of movements.

   b. Psychomotor agitation.

   c. Slowness of verbal response.

   d. Tremor.

5. Agitation as a manifestation of central (psychic) pain of severe depression in the setting of psychomotor retardation can be manifested as:

   a. Decreased speech latency.

   b. Hand wringing.

   c. Increased initiation of movements.

   d. Waxy flexibility.

See the testbank CD for more self-test questions.

5 CHAPTER

LABORATORY EVALUATIONS AND PSYCHOLOGICAL TESTING

Michael R. Privitera, MD, MS, and Jeffrey M. Lyness, MD

I. Laboratory Workup

A. Overview

  1. Broad range of medical and neurological conditions may contribute to psychopathology: includes rest of medicine
  2. Difficult to list all laboratory procedures used in psychiatric workup
  3. Clinical judgment, cost/benefit considerations, and standards of practice in community prevail
  4. Table 5.1 lists usual laboratory tests that may be considered for psychiatric patients

B. General guidelines

  1. Initial workup

   a. Direct clues from symptoms, history, physical exam, and known medical context drive decisions

> Example of range of workup: for a *healthy* 35-year-old with first-onset major depression of moderate severity, consider basic screening like complete blood count, electrolyte and glucose levels, and thyroid-stimulating hormone screen; however, a 35-year-old with known seropositivity for human immunodeficiency virus (HIV) who had the same depressive symptoms would require extensive laboratory evaluation, head neuroimaging, and possibly lumbar puncture.

TABLE 5.1

Laboratory Tests Commonly Considered to Evaluate Patients With Psychiatric Presentations*

General (Most Patients)	In Some Patient Populations (e.g., New-Onset in Older Patient) or Clinically as Indicated, Also Consider:
Complete blood count	Blood alcohol level
Electrolytes	Ceruloplasmin
Blood urea nitrogen	Heavy metal screen
Creatinine	Urinary or fecal porphyrins
Calcium	Thyroid antibodies
Hepatic enzymes	Neuroimaging (CT or MRI)
Thyroid-stimulating hormone	Electrocardiogram
Rapid plasma reagin (or venereal	Electroencephalogram
disease research lab) test	Chest x-ray
Erythrocyte sedimentation rate	Lumbar puncture
Vitamin B$_{12}$	
Folate	
Therapeutic drug levels	
Urinalysis	
Urine toxicology screen	

*Lab tests used for health monitoring while a patient is on psychotropic medication are beyond the scope of this table.

   b. Cognitive deficit disorder (e.g., delirium, dementia) by implication and definition has "organic" contributors and so requires laboratory workup; see Chapter 8
   c. If no worrisome medical history or cognitive deficit syndrome, consider following clinical criteria guide for laboratory evaluation (beyond normal health maintenance)
      i. New-onset psychiatric syndrome in elderly person
      ii. New-onset mania or psychosis, any age
      iii. New-onset anxiety or somatoform syndrome without psychiatric past history or personality disorder, age ≥ 30 years
      iv. "Personality change" in absence of Axis I disorder that could account for change
      v. Any psychiatric syndromes that fail to respond to usual treatments

vi. Recurrence of a disorder that is:
   (1) Not consistent with prior course
   (2) Not explained by:
      (A) Noncompliance
      (B) New psychosocial stressor
      (C) Other circumstances

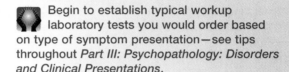

Begin to establish typical workup laboratory tests you would order based on type of symptom presentation—see tips throughout *Part III: Psychopathology: Disorders and Clinical Presentations.*

2. Laboratory monitoring **IV4**
   a. Therapeutic levels: drugs where therapeutic levels established (e.g., lithium, valproate, certain tricyclic antidepressants)
   b. Adverse side-effect/metabolism monitoring
      i. Clozapine: white blood count
      ii. Lithium: thyroid and kidney function
      iii. Valproate: liver function tests
      iv. Atypical antipsychotics: lipid, glucose metabolism, weight
      v. When suspected clinically

II. Psychological Testing
A. Overview
   1. Broad array of tests
      a. Administered by trained personnel
      b. Interview
      c. Pen, paper, and other means
   2. Doctorate-level psychologist needed to interpret results
   3. Classified (typed) by target of assessment
B. Types **IV3**
   1. Intelligence testing
      a. Measure global intellectual function
      b. Subscores focus on particular realms (e.g., Verbal Intelligence Quotient)
      c. Normed to general population
      d. 100 = mean; standard deviation defined at 15

TABLE 5.2	Terms for Clinically Significant Low IQ Scores
Severity	IQ Score Range
Borderline intellectual functioning	70–85
Mild mental retardation	50–55 to approximately 70
Moderate mental retardation	35–40 to 50–55
Severe mental retardation	20–25 to 35–40
Profound mental retardation	IQ below 20 or 25

See diagnostic criteria from DSM-IV-TR, American Psychiatric Association, 2000

    e. Score ranges define:
       i. Mental retardation
      ii. Superior function ("genius")
     iii. Table 5.2 lists scores used in Mental Retardation
          determination
2. Neuropsychological testing
    a. Assesses performance in specific cognitive realms
    b. May complement bedside cognitive testing
    c. May serve to document stability or changes in cognition
       over time
3. Personality testing
    a. Pen-and-paper tests
    b. Self-reported responses to questions that assess personality
       style and traits
    c. Current state of mind can influence response
    d. Considerable use in:
       i. Clinical research
      ii. Vocational assessments
     iii. Other applied psychology settings
    e. Usefulness limited in acute medical/psychiatric settings
4. Projective testing
    a. Asks patient to respond in open-ended and expansive manner
    b. Uses standardized stimuli
       i. Inkblots (Rorschach)
      ii. Drawings of evocative scenes (e.g., Thematic
          Apperception Test)
    c. Psychologists are trained to score these unstructured responses
       in structured ways to interpret results

d. Yields information on what may be prominent in patient's mental life but not obvious from clinical interview
  i. Themes
  ii. Conflicts
  iii. Affects
e. Not a substitute for diagnosis from clinical evaluation
f. May aid in diagnostic process revealing:
  i. Psychotic thought processes
  ii. Depressive themes
  iii. Other aspects not clearly evident otherwise

 MENTOR TIPS DIGEST

- Example of range of workup: for a *healthy* 35-year-old with first-onset major depression of moderate severity, consider basic screening like complete blood count, electrolyte and glucose levels, and thyroid-stimulating hormone screen; however, a 35-year-old with known seropositivity for HIV who had the same depressive symptoms would require extensive laboratory evaluation, head neuroimaging, and possibly lumbar puncture.
- Begin to establish typical workup laboratory tests you would order based on type of symptom presentation— see tips throughout *Part III: Psychopathology: Disorders and Clinical Presentations.*

Chapter Self-Test Questions

Circle the correct answer. After you have responded to the questions, check your answers in Appendix A.

1. Medical conditions that may contribute to psychopathology:

  a. Include only endocrinological conditions

  b. Include only neurological conditions

  c. Include the rest of the field of medicine

  d. Are rare

2. The decision to obtain laboratory workup for psychiatric patients over and above normal health maintenance should:

   a. Be based on clinical judgment, cost/benefit considerations, and standards of practice in community.

   b. Routinely include an electroencephalogram.

   c. Routinely include electrolytes and kidney function tests regardless of the details of the symptom presentation.

   d. Routinely include thyroid-stimulating hormone determination.

3. If there is no worrisome medical history, or no cognitive deficit syndrome exists, which of the following would be considered a reasonable guideline for obtaining laboratory evaluation in a psychiatric patient (beyond normal health maintenance)?

   a. A stereotypic personality change that occurs in a patient with recurrent depressive episodes

   b. New-onset psychiatric syndrome in an elderly person

   c. Recurrence of mania

   d. Recurrent psychotic episodes in a medication noncompliant patient who respond well to treatment

4. A psychotropic medication that has established and useful standardized therapeutic blood levels is:

   a. Haloperidol.

   b. Sertraline.

   c. Tranylcypromine.

   d. Valproate.

5. An antipsychotic drug whose adverse side effect of lowered white blood cell count needs to be routinely monitored is:

   a. Chlorpromazine.

   b. Clomipramine.

   c. Clonazepam.

   d. Clozapine.

See the testbank CD for more self-test questions.

DIAGNOSTIC IMPRESSION, FORMULATION, AND PLAN

Michael R. Privitera, MD, MS, and Jeffrey M. Lyness, MD

I. Overview

A. Every psychiatric workup ends with some kind of summation

B. Summation conveys:

    1. What you *think* about data you have gathered, organized, and presented

    2. What you *plan* to do from here

C. Commonly used format

    1. *Diagnostic impression* (list of diagnoses)

    2. *Formulation* (opportunity to discuss differential diagnostic thinking or consider etiological issues)

    3. *Plan* (description of what you are going to do)

D. Length of these sections (particularly Formulation and Plan) varies enormously depending on clinical setting

> Examples of range of lengths in Formulation section include an inpatient with a first psychotic presentation (would have significant details of differential diagnosis and etiological contributors) and an emergency room workup of an established psychiatric outpatient (shorter, with focus on presenting crisis and plans).

E. As a trainee, you may be asked to write more complete summations than needed otherwise.

    1. To further your learning

    2. To demonstrate to your teachers what you know and how you think about clinical situations at hand

> Ask your preceptors about their expectations about length, format, and amount of detail in differential diagnosis discussion in Formulation. When writing Plan section, review with your preceptor how she/he wants you to demonstrate your thinking, i.e., what goes in chart before or after they review it, what does not go in chart and may be for eyes and ears of your preceptor only.

II. Recording Your Diagnostic Impression

  A. Diagnostic reasoning in psychiatry `II 1-3`

    1. Multiaxial System format of *Diagnostic and Statistical Manual of Mental Disorders* (DSM-IV-TR)

      a. Each axis refers to a different *domain* of clinical information

      b. Is comprehensive and systematic

      c. Captures complexity of clinical situations

      d. Promotes Biopsychosocial Model

      e. Table 6.1 explains multiaxial assessment

    2. Axis I

      a. Most psychiatric diagnoses go here, principal diagnosis listed first

      b. Other conditions that may be focus of clinical attention (important conditions that do not count as true mental disorder, e.g., normal bereavement)

      c. Rule-outs (e.g., "X" versus "Y")

TABLE 6.1

Multiaxial Assessment `ADMSEP II 3`	
Axis	**What it Covers**
I	Most psychiatric disorders Other conditions that may be a focus of clinical attention
II	Personality disorders Mental Retardation
III	General Medical Conditions
IV	Psychosocial and environmental problems
V	Global Assessment of Functioning (GAF)

For details, see American Psychiatric Association: Diagnostic and Statistical Manual of Mental Disorders, 4th ed, Text Revision. Washington DC, American Psychiatric Association, 2000.

3. Axis II
   a. Includes rule-outs when applicable
   b. "Deferred" if information available too scant to suggest presence or absence
   c. If data point to presence or absence of personality pathology, then say so
   d. Put "(Principal Diagnosis)" after diagnosis if main reason for visit
4. Axis III
   a. List of medical illnesses should include rule-outs or differential when appropriate
   b. Diagnoses that cause cognitive or secondary psychiatric disorders should be included on Axis I (e.g., "mood disorder, depressed due to hypothyroidism")
5. Axis IV
   a. Stressful life events (referred to as *stressors*)
   b. Ongoing problematic environmental issues (in patient's psychosocial milieu)
6. Axis V
   a. Number from 0 to 100, reflecting your estimate of patient's level of functioning
   b. Based upon psychiatric issues only, not physical limitations
   c. Use anchor points in the DSM-IV Global Assessment of Functioning (GAF) scale
   d. Score *current* GAF and *baseline* GAF (highest functioning in last 1 year)

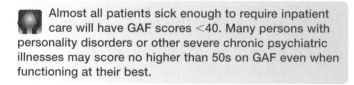 Almost all patients sick enough to require inpatient care will have GAF scores <40. Many persons with personality disorders or other severe chronic psychiatric illnesses may score no higher than 50s on GAF even when functioning at their best.

   e. Table 6.2 provides a sample multiaxial assessment.

III. Recording Your Formulation
   A. Differential diagnosis
      1. Avoid premature closure; important in psychiatry as in other fields of medicine
         a. Treatment dictated by accurate diagnosis

TABLE 6.2

Sample Multiaxial Assessment

Axis	Sample Assessment
I	Major Depressive Disorder vs. Alcohol-Induced Mood Disorder, Depressed Type vs. Mood Disorder due to antihypertensive medications Alcohol Dependence Rule out Social Phobia
II	Rule out Avoidant Personality Disorder
III	Asthma, stable Essential Hypertension
IV	Separation from spouse Decrease in income due to job layoff
V	Current GAF: 35–40 High GAF in past year: 65–70

   2. How do patient's symptoms cluster together into recognizable syndrome? **II 4–5**
   3. How do these syndromes fit into particular disorders?

> In Differential Diagnosis section, defend your reasoning. For example, explain why you think the psychotic syndrome is caused by medication toxicity rather than a primary psychotic disorder; or explain why you believe prominent anxiety symptoms are part of a major depressive illness rather than a primary anxiety disorder.

   4. Table 6.3 provides a symptom-driven guide to differential diagnosis.
   5. If diagnoses are still unclear, what specific data do you need to clarify them?
      a. Observations about symptoms over time?
      b. Recent observations by other informants?
      c. Old records describing previous episodes?
   B. Indicate focal problem that you have identified, i.e., why is patient presenting *now*?

TABLE 6.3	
Symptom-Driven Guide to Differential Diagnosis	
Symptom	Can Occur In
Anorexia	Anorexia Nervosa Depressive Disorder NOS Dysthymia General Medical Conditions Major Depressive Episode

Anxiety	Acute Stress Disorder
	Adjustment Disorder with Anxious Mood
	Agoraphobia
	Anxiety Disorder NOS
	Anxiety due to General Medical
	    Conditions
	Associated feature of many other mental
	    disorders (Body Dysmorphic Disorder,
	    Dysthymia, Major Depression,
	    Schizophrenia)
	Delusional Disorders
	Generalized Anxiety Disorder
	Obsessive Compulsive Disorder
	Panic attacks
	Panic Disorder
	Personality Disorders
	Post Traumatic Stress Disorder
	Realistic concerns
	Separation Anxiety Disorder
	Social Phobia
	Specific Phobia
	Substance Induced
	Substance Withdrawal

Attention difficulties	Anxiety Disorder
	Attention Deficit/Hyperactivity Disorder
	Dissociative Disorder
	Mood Disorders: Major Depressive,
	    Hypomanic, and Manic Episodes
	Personality Change due to General Medical
	    Conditions
	Personality Disorder

(continued on page 74)

TABLE 6.3	Symptom-Driven Guide to Differential Diagnosis (continued)
Symptom	**Can Occur In**
	Pervasive Developmental Disorder
	Psychotic Disorder
	Substance Related Disorder
Depressed mood	Adjustment Disorder with Depressed Mood
	Bereavement
	Cyclothymic Disorder
	Delirium (often hypoactive type)
	Dementia
	Depressive Disorder NOS
	Dysthymic Disorder
	Major Depressive Episode
	Mixed Episode
	Mood Disorder due to General Medical Condition
	Normal sadness
	Schizoaffective Disorder, Depressed and Bipolar types
	Substance Induced Mood Disorder
Excessive activity/impulsive behavior/euphoria	Antidepressant Induced
	Bipolar Disorder NOS
	Cyclothymic Disorder
	Delirium
	ECT Induced
	Hyperactivity in ADHD (no euphoria)
	Hypomanic Episode
	Light Therapy Induced
	Manic Episode
	Mixed Episodes
	Mood Disorder due to General Medical Condition
	Substance Induced Mood Disorder
Obsessive/ ruminative thinking *May have true obsessions	Anxiety Disorder due to General Medical Condition*
	Body Dysmorphic Disorder
	Delusional Disorder

Symptom-Driven Guide to Differential Diagnosis (continued)

Symptom	Can Occur In
	Eating Disorder
	Generalized Anxiety Disorder
	Hypochondriasis*
	Major Depressive Episode
	Obsessive Compulsive Disorder*
	Obsessive Compulsive Personality Disorder
	Paraphilias
	Pathological Gambling
	Psychotic Disorder NOS
	Schizophrenia
	Social Phobia
	Specific Phobia
	Substance Abuse
	Substance Induced Anxiety Disorder*
	Superstitions*
Psychosis# **#Psychosis may be manifested by hallucinations, delusions, or thought process derailments.**	Body Dysmorphic Disorder
	Brief Psychotic Disorder
	Delirium
	Delusional Disorder
	Dementia
	Major Depressive Episode (with Psychotic Features)
	Manic Episode
	Psychotic Disorder NOS
	Schizoaffective Disorder
	Schizophrenia
	Substance Induced (e.g., cocaine, amphetamines)

1. Usual focal problems for inpatient admissions
   a. Suicidal ideation
   b. Homicidal ideation
   c. Severe functional incapacity
2. For new outpatient evaluations
   a. Less severe suicidal ideation
   b. Less severe homicidal ideation
   c. Less severe functional incapacity

 d. Specific target symptoms ("I'm feeling depressed")
 e. Behaviors ("My wife and I are arguing too much")
 3. Ongoing cases
   a. More difficult to reduce to a single focal problem
   b. Still important to identify and prioritize goals of treatment
     i. Short-term goals
     ii. Long-term goals
 C. How do you *understand* patient's diagnoses and focal problem?
   1. If more than one diagnosis, how do they influence each other?
   2. How is focal problem tied to psychiatric diagnoses?
   3. How are focal problem and psychiatric diagnoses related to, or explainable, by the following?
     a. Current psychosocial factors (e.g., family dynamics or stressful life events)
     b. Psychodynamic formulation of patient

> Psychodynamic formulation refers to an appraisal of salient conflicts, usual defense mechanisms, and interpersonal relatedness, along with analysis of how/if these are related to current presentation and treatment implementation; this may include a developmental perspective on current psychodynamic issues.

     c. Other psychological perspectives (e.g., learning theory, cognitive psychology)
     d. Genetic factors
     e. Neurobiological alterations or mechanisms
     f. General medical conditions, medications, and other physiological factors
     g. Mechanisms by which treatments may help the presenting problem(s)

IV. Recording Your Plan II-8
 A. Organize plans by a problem list (just as you have done in general medical settings).
 B. Psychiatric presentation may be encompassed under one item ("psychiatric") or via several different items (especially if multiple diagnoses or complex psychosocial issues).

For patients with multiple diagnoses or complex psychosocial issues, consider listing items such as "family discord" or "social isolation" as separate problems needing to be addressed.

C. List and address all medical problems.
D. For each problem describe what you will do and with what aim: "Begin nortriptyline to target major depressive syndrome," "Address cognitive depressive distortions in cognitive/psychoeducational individual psychotherapy," or "Family meeting to discuss psycho-education, sources of conflict with patient, and resources available after discharge from hospital."
E. Ends with discussion about overall expectations for course of treatment.

 Examples of overall expectations that would apply for inpatient or partial hospital admissions:

1. What is expected length of stay?
2. What is expected disposition plan?
3. Outpatients: how long seen, how will end of treatment be determined?

MENTOR TIPS DIGEST

- Examples of range of lengths in Formulation section include an inpatient with a first psychotic presentation (would have significant details of differential diagnosis and etiologic contributors) to emergency room workup of established psychiatric outpatient (shorter, with focus on presenting crisis and plans).
- Ask your preceptors about their expectations about length, format, and amount of detail in differential diagnosis discussion in Formulation. When writing Plan section, review with your preceptor how they want you to demonstrate your thinking, i.e., what goes in chart before or after they review it, what does not go in chart and may be for eyes and ears of your preceptor only.

- Almost all patients sick enough to require inpatient care will have GAF scores <40. Many persons with personality disorders or other severe chronic psychiatric illnesses may score no higher than 50s on GAF even when functioning at their best.
- In Differential Diagnosis section, defend your reasoning. For example, explain why you think the psychotic syndrome is caused by medication toxicity rather than a primary psychotic disorder; or explain why you believe prominent anxiety symptoms are part of a major depressive illness rather than a primary anxiety disorder.
- Psychodynamic formulation refers to an appraisal of salient conflicts, usual defense mechanisms, and interpersonal relatedness, along with analysis of how/if these are related to current presentation and treatment implementation; this may include a developmental perspective on current psychodynamic issues.
- For patients with multiple diagnoses or complex psychosocial issues, consider listing items such as "family discord" or "social isolation" as separate problems needing to be addressed.
- Examples of overall expectations that would apply for inpatient or partial hospital admissions: (1) What is expected length of stay? (2) What is expected disposition plan? and (3) Outpatients: how long seen, and how will end of treatment be determined?

Chapter Self-Test Questions

Circle the correct answer. After you have responded to the questions, check your answers in Appendix A.

1. The summation at the end of a psychiatric workup conveys what you *think* about data that you have gathered, organized, and presented, and what other major component?
   a. Laboratory data
   b. Mental Status Examination
   c. Source of the patient referral
   d. What you *plan* to do from here

2. The major reasons that as a trainee you are asked to write more complete summations than may be needed otherwise are to further your learning, demonstrate to your teachers what you know, and:

   a. Continue the tradition in training.

   b. Demonstrate how you think about clinical situations at hand.

   c. Ensure that you spend sufficient time on the patient.

   d. Ensure you include excessive detail so that others may know in the future.

3. Each axis in the Multiaxial System format of *Diagnostic and Statistical Manual of Mental Disorder* (DSM) refers to a:

   a. Different domain of clinical information.

   b. Length of time of each symptom.

   c. Major stressor involved in the clinical presentation.

   d. Treatment plan for each symptom that occurs.

4. In a Multiaxial System format of diagnoses, Axis II lists Personality Disorders and:

   a. General medical conditions.

   b. Global assessment of functioning.

   c. Mental Retardation.

   d. Psychosocial and environmental problems.

5. Diagnoses that cause cognitive or secondary psychiatric disorders should be listed on:

   a. Axis I.

   b. Axis III.

   c. Axis IV.

   d. Axis V.

See the testbank CD for more self-test questions.

three

PSYCHOPATHOLOGY: DISORDERS AND CLINICAL PRESENTATIONS

7

PSYCHIATRIC EMERGENCIES AND URGENT CARE ISSUES

**Michael R. Privitera, MD, MS, and
Jeffrey M. Lyness, MD**

I. Suicide
  A. Overview
    1. Suicidality exists on a continuum of self-destructive behaviors
    (Table 7.1)
      a. Chronic acts that ultimately prove harmful

TABLE 7.1

Self-Destructive Acts and Suicide (ADMSEP V 1-2)		
Example	**Time Frame**	**Common Intentions**
1) Poor health choice(s) (e.g., cigarette smoking)	Chronic	Immediate gratification Ultimately harmful Intentions vary: not care/immediate gratification–centered/ eventual harm Long-term death gamble*
2) Self-injurious behavior (SIB) (e.g., cutting self superficially, hand or head banging)	Acute/ subacute/ chronic	Usually relief of psychic pain and/or self-loathing (i.e., self-punishment) Some may get euphoria Sometimes mixed self-harm and death gamble Psychotic patients may do so to maintain contact with reality
3) Sublethal attempt and *knows* sublethal method	Acute	Multiple interpersonal Spectrum from no intention to die to death gamble Attempts to change environment of relationship(s) in some way or avoid consequences (e.g., prison)
4) Lethal attempt but *thought* it was a *sublethal* method	Acute	Similar to 3) Can die by mistake

Increasing acuteness of lethality risk →

Self-Destructive Acts and Suicide ADMSEP V 1-2 (continued)

Example	Time Frame	Common Intentions
5) Sublethal attempt but *thought* it was a *lethal* method	Acute	Death (Watch very carefully as next time may find method that is lethal)
6) Lethal attempt and *thought* it was a *lethal* method	Acute	Death

*Death gamble: taking a chance (gamble), with attitude of "maybe it will kill me, or maybe it won't"

    b. Acute acts that are physically harmful without intent or potential for death

    c. Acute acts with clear intent or potential for killing oneself

2. Suicide "gesture": term sometimes used to refer to suicide attempts of low lethality

> Beware of the term suicide "gesture"; this term sometimes says as much about our own reaction to the attempt (and attempter) as it does about the objective reality of the event.

> Examples of low-lethality suicide attempts include superficial cutting and burning (e.g., with lit cigarette) or swallowing objects (e.g., tacks, paper clips). V 1-2

    a. Sometimes motive is external and obvious (e.g., avoiding prison)

    b. Some patients describe these acts as means of relieving tension or anxiety (without intent to die)

    c. Occasionally, psychotic patients use such behaviors to try to maintain contact with reality (pain or wound—from real world—distracts from internal psychotic preoccupations)

3. Motives may be difficult to discern reliably

4. Self-destructive acts should *always* be taken seriously

B. Clinical risk factors

  1. Suicide attempters and those who die by suicide are different, if overlapping, populations

  2. Some risk factors and clinical characteristics are similar, others quite different

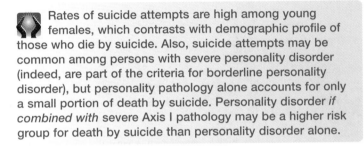

Rates of suicide attempts are high among young females, which contrasts with demographic profile of those who die by suicide. Also, suicide attempts may be common among persons with severe personality disorder (indeed, are part of the criteria for borderline personality disorder), but personality pathology alone accounts for only a small portion of death by suicide. Personality disorder *if combined with* severe Axis I pathology may be a higher risk group for death by suicide than personality disorder alone.

  3. Factors related to *death by suicide* `V 1-2`

    a. Older age

      i. Suicide in adolescents gets far more media attention

        (1) Adolescent suicide rates are rising

        (2) Suicide is one of the top causes of death in this age group

      ii. Suicide rates are much higher in elderly

        (1) Greater frailty

        (2) More likely to use highly lethal means

          (A) Ratio of suicide to attempted suicide higher in elderly than younger people

    b. Male gender

      i. Males of all ages are more likely to use violent and lethal means (raising rate of death by suicide)

    c. White race

      i. In United States, whites more likely than other ethnicities (may reflect complex combination of factors)

    d. Other demographic and cultural factors

      i. Rates vary greatly across religious groups, nationalities, and other cultural markers

      ii. Living alone

iii. Widowed, divorced, or separated marital status

    iv. Unemployment or retired work status

        (1) These latter factors may contribute to suicide directly or as manifestations of clinical conditions that predispose to suicide

  e. Psychiatric diagnoses

    i. Most but not all persons who kill themselves have diagnosable psychiatric disorder at time of their death

    ii. Most common

        (1) Chronic psychotic disorders

           (A) Schizophrenia

           (B) Schizoaffective disorder

        (2) Substance-use disorders

           (A) Especially alcohol dependence

        (3) Mood disorders

           (A) Mostly major depression

> In suicidal elderly, mood disorders clearly predominate among those with a diagnosable condition.

  f. Stressors

    i. Common events or themes

        (1) Interpersonal losses

        (2) Other losses

        (3) Medical illnesses (actual and perceived)

        (4) Family discord

  g. Personality

    i. DSM-IV-TR personality disorders of limited usefulness in predicting suicide

    ii. Empirical research: supports clinical notions that suicidal persons have rigid, inflexible, or otherwise limited coping mechanisms, particularly in approach to problem solving

C. Additional perspectives on suicidal behavior

  1. Attempts to understand biopsychosocial pathophysiology of suicidal behavior draw on numerous levels of conceptual organization.

  2. All may play some role, although predominant factors may vary among different suicidal people.

3. The breadth and depth of the field of suicidology is greater than what can be contained in this chapter.

4. Beyond theories involving personality, stressors, cultural factors, other social factors, and biopsychosocial concomitants of gender and age, three other additional overlapping perspectives are worth highlighting

   a. There may be genetics, neurobiology, and neuroendocrinology of suicide that cut across psychiatric diagnostic boundaries; e.g., suicidal persons may have decreased activity of serotonergic systems, analogous to (but independent of) the decrease seen in depression.

   b. Suicidal behavior may have any of several overt or unconscious "goals," including expressions of:

      i. Despair (desire to remove oneself from environment).

      ii. Rage (desire to express anger or exact punishment on others).

      iii. Help seeking (desire to change behavior of others to get one's needs met).

   c. In some cases, suicidality may be helpfully understood as nothing more or less than a symptom of an acute Axis I disorder (which will remit when the acute episode remits)

      i. Although this perspective does not always apply, may be useful in many clinical situations

D. Assessment

   1. In assessing suicidality, consider the following factors

      a. Demographic and clinical risk factors listed previously

      b. Explicit delineation of patient's ideation, plans, intent (as discussed in Chapter 4)

      c. Details of the attempt itself

         i. Extent of advanced preparations (such as completion of a will, shifting bank accounts for one's heirs, and so forth)

         ii. Precautions taken to preclude discovery

         iii. Lethality of the method

   2. It is important to be humble about our ability to predict suicide, which is extraordinarily complexly-determined behavior

      a. It is a relatively unlikely outcome in any single given situation.

         i. Most sophisticated attempts to develop predictive algorithms (using as rich a database as possible) have failed to predict suicide enough to be clinically helpful.

b. We do know much with which to inform our clinical judgment—yet *judgment* part remains.

II. Violence
A. Overview
1. Violence is increasingly prominent and problematic part of society
2. Neurobiological, psychological, and social sciences can help us understand violence better than psychiatry per se
3. Psychiatry (medical specialty of diagnosing and treating mental disorder) as regards to violence
   a. Can offer only limited insights
   b. Even more limited in ability to predict or prevent specific acts of violence
4. Much of psychiatric assessment of patients for violence overlaps with assessments discussed previously
5. Larger consideration of violent behavior, although beyond scope of this book, is extremely important: e.g., screening for child abuse, adult domestic violence, rape, and elder abuse **V 11–14**
6. What follows are additional pointers with your work in clinical settings
B. Clinical risk factors **V 6–7**
1. Clinical guides rather than statements about absolute risk
2. In community, risk of violence
   a. Psychotic patients ≈ general population
3. In psychiatric or other patient care settings
4. Psychosis may lead to violence and worth noting in clinical assessment
5. Clinical guides
   a. Male gender
   b. Prior history of violence
   c. Prior history of, or current evidence for, other types of poor impulse control
   d. Psychiatric diagnosis or acute state including:
      i. Mania (may be single best predictor of violence in psychiatric inpatient settings)
      ii. Psychosis
      iii. Substance-related states
         (1) Intoxication
         (2) Withdrawal

iv. Cognitive impairments
  (1) Delirium
  (2) Dementia
  (3) Mental retardation
v. Personality disorders
  (1) Especially those marked by chronic difficulties with impulse control
    (A) Borderline Personality Disorder
    (B) Antisocial Personality Disorder
    (C) Other personality disorder when acute stressor and sense of losing control or feeling overwhelmed
vi. Depression (if comorbid with any of above)

C. Management of violence or imminent violence **V 7-8**

1. First ensure your safety and (within reason) comfort.
  a. You cannot help your patient unless you are able to use your skills and mental resources freely and effectively.
  b. Set limits on a threatening situation.
  c. Get out of the situation if setting limits is not possible or effective.
  d. Get additional help (staff, security, police) sooner rather than later, if necessary.

2. Verbal interventions that may help defuse a potentially violent patient walk a line between: **V 9**
  a. Helping patient feel empowered and understood (which may make him or her feel calmer and less prone to be violent) and
  b. Setting limits on unacceptable behavior

> To set limits in a violent or imminently violent situation, comments such as "I'm not going to be able to help you unless you stop threatening me" or "I need to ask you to sit down and stop waving your fists in the air" may be entirely appropriate.

3. When patients are actually violent or losing control of their physical impulses, a "psychiatric code" is instituted.
  a. *Marshalling sufficient forces* (usually psychiatric staff plus security personnel) to meet needs of situation—enough for safety, and with potential "show of force" that may help the patient get back into control

b. *Deciding on a specific plan of action* that is understood by entire code team

> Possible scenario of psychiatric code plan of action: "We're going to put the patient into four-point leather restraints on this stretcher bed and then administer an IM injection of lorazepam (Ativan) 2 mg." At this time it is important that specific roles be assigned to each team member: "You will restrain the patient's left leg, I will give the injection" **V7**

c. *Implementing the plan*, during which time main verbal contact with patient (usually one person takes this role) will consist of *what* will be done to him or her; explanation of *whys* or answers to patient question must await completion of code when patient and staff are presumably safe from harm

> During implementation of psychiatric code plan (within the bounds of your own and patient's safety), remember patient respect and opportunities for patient to still save face by offering choices possible.

III. Psychological Trauma
A. Psychiatric consequences of exposure to life-threatening or otherwise unusually horrific situation
B. After experiencing events such as rapes, beatings, or physical disasters, persons vary widely in their responses **V13**
 1. Depression
 2. Post-traumatic stress disorder
 3. Acute stress disorder
 4. Mania
 5. Psychosis
 6. Anxiety
 7. Somatoform disorders
 8. No diagnosable syndrome at all
C. Approach to patient with recent trauma must vary, depending on details of event and context

D. Common principles learned from research and clinical experience (from combat soldiers; victims of earthquakes, floods, and other natural disasters; and victims of rape) to reduce acute symptoms and probably long-term complications as well **V 14**

  1. Immediate use of brief psychotherapeutic techniques

    a. Building an alliance

    b. Empathy

    c. Support

    d. Validating

    e. Encouraging expression of thoughts and affects

  2. Inform patients about availability of ongoing psychiatric services and other relevant supports

IV. Catatonia

A. Overview

  1. Syndrome characterized by:

    a. Severe psychomotor abnormality, which may include:

      i. Purposeless, self-directed, increased motor activity

      ii. Severe slowing or immobility; latter may include catalepsy (a.k.a. "waxy flexibility," in which limb position may be "molded" by the examiner, and patient maintains this position)

      iii. Peculiar voluntary movements, including bizarre posturing, stereotypes, or other prominent mannerisms

    b. Mutism

    c. Negativism (resistance to all instruction or attempts at being moved)

    d. Echolalia (repeating others' phrases) or echopraxia (mimicking others' postures or movements)

B. Assessment

  1. Differential diagnosis of catatonia includes:

    a. Variety of neurological conditions (e.g., encephalitis, vascular events, Parkinson's disease)

    b. Systemic conditions, most typically metabolic (e.g., hepatic failure, electrolyte disturbances)

    c. Medication side effects (e.g., neuroleptics)

    d. Idiopathic mood disorders (bipolar disorder, major depression)

    e. Schizophrenia

    f. Schizoaffective Disorder

> In patients newly presenting with catatonia, it may be difficult or impossible to tell whether delirium is also present. How can cognitive impairment, the hallmark of delirium, be assessed in a patient who is mute or resistant to commands and questions? Therefore, catatonia, like delirium, must be treated as a medical emergency until proved otherwise. **V3**

C. Management of idiopathic catatonia
   1. Assuming medical workup failed to identify a specific cause, proceed to treat as if idiopathic psychiatric disorder.
   2. Most people with de novo idiopathic catatonia ultimately turn out to have mood disorder (bipolar or unipolar) with psychotic features
   3. Careful history of symptoms apparent *prior to* full catatonic state, as well as patient's past psychiatric and family history, may be helpful
   4. Keys to management include:
      a. Supportive care
         i. Nasogastric or intravenous access to maintain adequate hydration and nutrition
         ii. Monitoring vital signs
         iii. Care related to bladder and bowel function
         iv. Attempts to prevent deconditioning by passive or active exercise
      b. Benzodiazepines
         i. Oral or parenteral (best described for lorazepam) may rapidly "lyse" catatonic state
         ii. Underlying affective or psychotic condition remains, but supportive care and engagement with treatment often are much easier (e.g., may now take fluids, food, oral medications)
      c. Other drugs
         i. Neuroleptics, mood stabilizers, or antidepressants may be needed per underlying episode or overall illness
      d. Electroconvulsive therapy (ECT)
         i. Rapidity and great efficacy for mood episodes with psychotic features
         ii. May be first choice

iii. Obtaining informed consent from a catatonic patient may be obstacle to its use

iv. State laws vary: in some places, informed consent from next of kin may be used

V. Medical Emergencies of Direct Relevance to Psychiatry

A. Overview

1. Common emergencies related to psychiatric disorders
2. Physical trauma (including self-inflicted wounds)
3. Physical sequelae of substance intoxication or withdrawal
4. Intentional overdoses and self-poisonings
5. Medical emergencies related to psychotropic medications: three are reviewed below

B. Acute Dystonic Reaction V 5

1. Side effects of dystonia on the antipsychotic drug type called neuroleptics are reviewed in Chapter 16.
2. It is useful to remember that other dopamine blockers are not usually thought of as neuroleptics, such as prochlorperazine (Compazine) and metoclopramide (Reglan), may also cause dystonia.
3. Severe acute dystonia occurs most often in younger people, especially men.
4. Dramatic, uncomfortable, and potentially dangerous presentations may include:
   a. Torticollis (neck spasms).
   b. Opisthotonos (severe extension of entire spine).
   c. Oculogyric crisis (fixed upward gaze).
   d. Laryngeal dystonia, which may lead to upper airway obstruction.
5. Treatment
   a. Intramuscular anticholinergics (e.g., benztropine [Cogentin]) or diphenhydramine (Benadryl) usually leads to rapid relief.
   b. Use supportive measures, including securing adequate airway in case of laryngeal dystonia, until pharmacological relief is obtained.

> In treating acute dystonic reaction, remember to order oral doses of anticholinergic/diphenhydramine to follow intramuscular rescue. Half-life of neuroleptic drug may be longer than anticholinergic, and dystonic reaction may otherwise come back again in a few hours.

C. Neuroleptic Malignant Syndrome (NMS)
  1. Potentially fatal idiosyncratic reaction to traditional, but sometimes atypical, neuroleptic drugs
  2. Probably exists along a broad spectrum of severity
  3. In full-blown form includes the following symptoms
     a. Extrapyramidal side effects, especially rigidity
     b. Fever (may be quite high)
     c. Autonomic instability
        i. Diaphoresis
        ii. Wide fluctuations between low and high blood pressure, heart rate variability
        iii. Arrhythmias
     d. Delirium
     e. Seizures
     f. Skeletal muscle breakdown (due to severe rigidity), causing elevated serum creatine kinase levels
     g. Renal failure (due to myoglobinemia or hypoperfusion)
     h. Death (due to cardiovascular collapse, respiratory compromise, or renal failure)
  4. Treatment of NMS
     a. Discontinuation of all neuroleptic drugs and other dopamine blockers
     b. Supportive care: hydration; cooling blankets; monitoring and management of cardiac, cardiovascular, and respiratory function; monitoring of renal function and dialysis when indicated; anticonvulsants
     c. Dantrolene: muscle relaxant, may help with rigidity and consequent muscle breakdown
     d. Bromocriptine: central dopamine agonist, may help neurological components of NMS syndrome
  5. Anecdotal evidence suggests patients with resolved NMS may tolerate alternative neuroleptic drugs, usually an agent from a different chemical class
     a. Weigh risks of using alternative agent versus not using neuroleptic at all
D. Serotonin Syndrome
  1. Uncommon but potentially life-threatening
  2. Associated with drugs that potentiate serotonin in the central nervous system (CNS)

3. Onset usually within 24 hours, usually within 6 hours of initiation of drug or change in dosing

4. In full-blown form, has following symptoms

   a. Autonomic: hypertension, hypotension, tachycardia, diaphoreses, shivering, sialorrhea, mydriasis, tachypnea

   b. Behavioral: restlessness, agitation

   c. Gastrointestinal: nausea, vomiting, diarrhea, incontinence

   d. Hyperthermia (associated with more life-threatening outcome)

   e. Mental status: delirium, confusion, anxiety, irritability, euphoria, dysphoria, hallucinations

   f. Neurological: ataxia/incoordination, tremor, myoclonus, hyperflexia, ankle clonus, variable muscle rigidity (mild if present)

   g. Complications: rhabdomyolysis, renal failure, disseminated intravascular coagulation

> Serotonin Syndrome may at times be difficult to distinguish from NMS. Shivering, diarrhea (GI symptoms), tremor, hyperreflexia, and myoclonus tend to point more toward Serotonin Syndrome. Rigidity and very high creatine phosphokinase (CPK) levels tend to point more toward NMS. Table 7.2 compares and contrasts Serotonin Syndrome and NMS.

E. Selective Serotonin Reuptake Inhibitor (SSRI) Discontinuation Syndrome

   1. Occurs with abrupt discontinuation, or too rapid taper of SSRI or Serotonin Noradrenaline Reuptake Inhibitor (SNRI) antidepressants

   2. Onset typically 2–4 days

   3. Lasts up to 21 days

   4. Theoretical etiology: sudden absence of blockade of reuptake pump causes influx of neurotransmitter into presynaptic cell, depleting synapse of neurotransmitter

   5. Symptoms

     a. Somatic: dizziness, lightheadedness, nausea, vomiting, fatigue, lethargy, myalgia, chills and other flu-like symptoms, sensory and sleep disturbances

     b. Psychological: anxiety and/or agitation, crying spells, irritability, lowered mood

TABLE 7.2		
Comparison of Serotonin Syndrome and Neuroleptic Malignant Syndrome ADMSEP V 3-5		
Serotonin Syndrome		Neuroleptic Malignant Syndrome
Drugs that enhance serotonin in CNS	**Setting**	Neuroleptic use, or dopamine withdrawal
≤24 h of initiation or dose change	**Onset**	Days to weeks
<24 h to days (depends on T^1/$_2$ of drug)	**Resolution**	Average is 9 days
Delirium Confusion Dysphoria Irritability Euphoria Anxiety Hallucinations	**Cognitive**	Delirium
Restlessness Agitation	**Behavioral**	Muteness Sometime restlessness Sometime agitation
Fever BP instability Diaphoresis **Shivering*** **Diarrhea***	**Autonomic**	Fever BP instability Diaphoresis Tachycardia Tachypnea
Neuromuscular hyperreactivity **Tremor*** **Hyperreflexia*** **Myoclonus*** Ataxia/incoordination	**Neuromuscular**	Sluggish neuromuscular response **Rigidity*** Bradyreflexia Movement disorder
Uncommon, may have, but usually not severe Increased CPK Increased white blood cell (WBC) count	**Laboratory**	**Markedly increased CPK levels (usually >1000 IU/L; can go as high as 100,000 IU/L)*** Increased WBC count Increased LFT values

(continued on page 96)

TABLE 7.2		
Comparison of Serotonin Syndrome and Neuroleptic Malignant Syndrome ADMSEP V 3–5 **(continued)**		
Serotonin Syndrome		**Neuroleptic Malignant Syndrome**
Increased liver function test (LFT) values		
Discontinue (D/C) offending medication; wait	**Treatment**	D/C offending medication
Supportive measures		Supportive measures
Methysergide (5-HT antagonist)		Dantrolene (muscle relaxant)
Cyproheptadine (5-HT antagonist)		Bromocriptine (dopamine agonist)
Propranolol (5-HT 1A antagonist)		Amantadine (dopamine agonist)

* = Most important distinguishing features for each diagnosis

 SSRI Discontinuation Syndrome mnemonic:
AMINES:
A → Adrenergic excess symptoms
M → Mood fluctuations
IN → Intestinal flu-like illness
E → Extrapyramidal symptoms
S → Sleep disturbances

6. Virtual exception: fluoxetine, as half-life is long, and active metabolite has very long half-life (9 days)
7. Treatment
   a. Reinstitution of drug
   b. Taper more slowly
   c. Switching to other antidepressant of similar action usually works quickly, unless discontinued drug is high risk for syndrome and therefore may also require taper of first drug

d. Consider switch to or addition of fluoxetine at end of taper paradigm (to embed a slower taper of SSRI by its long half-life)

e. In medical settings, where patient not able to take medications by mouth, consider IV lorazepam (target is anxiety) and IV anticholinergics (target is cholinergic excess symptoms)

> To distinguish SSRI Discontinuation Syndrome from recurrence of Major Depressive Episode, consider the following when reinstituting SSRI:
> If relief is in hours—think SSRI Discontinuation Syndrome.
> If relief takes several days to weeks—think recurrence of Major Depressive Episode.

F. Tyramine-Induced Hypertensive Crisis
  1. May be consequence of straying from low tyramine diet or contraindicated medications (e.g., sympathomimetic amines) while patient on monoamine oxidase inhibitor (MAOI) antidepressant
  2. See Chapter 16 for more details on symptoms of such a crisis
  3. Main treatment strategy is control of malignant hypertension
     a. Some physicians routinely give prescription for nifedipine 10 mg capsules and how to administer in case of crisis
     b. Emergency room setting
        i. Standard procedures for reducing blood pressure
        ii. In addition, intravenous *alpha-adrenergic blockers* may be particularly effective (much of hypertension due to vasoconstriction from release of endogenous sympathomimetic drugs).
           (1) Phentolamine (excellent)
           (2) Chlorpromazine (also used)

MENTOR TIPS DIGEST

- Beware of the term suicide "gesture", this term sometimes says as much about our own reaction to the attempt (and attempter) as it does about the objective reality of the event.

- Examples of low-lethality suicide attempts include superficial cutting and burning (e.g., with lit cigarette) or swallowing objects (e.g., tacks, paper clips).
- Rates of suicide attempts are high among young females, which contrasts with demographic profile of those who die by suicide Also, suicide attempts may be common among persons with severe personality disorder (indeed are part of the criteria for borderline personality disorder), but personality pathology alone accounts for only a small portion of death by suicide. Personality Disorder *if combined with* severe Axis I pathology may be a higher risk group for death by suicide than personality disorder alone.
- In suicidal elderly, mood disorders clearly predominate among those with a diagnosable condition.
- To set limits in a violent or imminently violent situation, comments such as "I'm not going to be able to help you unless you stop threatening me" or "I need to ask you to sit down and stop waving your fists in the air" may be entirely appropriate.
- Possible scenario of psychiatric code plan of action: "We're going to put the patient into four-point leather restraints on this stretcher bed and then administer an IM injection of lorazepam (Ativan) 2 mg." At this time it is important that specific roles be assigned to each team member: "You will restrain the patient's left leg, I will give the injection."
- During implementation of psychiatric code plan (within the bounds of your own and patient's safety), remember patient respect and opportunities for patient to still save face by offering choices possible.
- In patients newly presenting with catatonia, it may be difficult or impossible to tell whether delirium is also present. How can cognitive impairment, the hallmark of delirium, be assessed in a patient who is mute or resistant to commands and questions? Therefore, catatonia, like delirium, must be treated as a medical emergency until proved otherwise.
- In treating acute dystonic reaction, order oral doses of anticholinergic/diphenhydramine to follow intramuscular rescue. Half-life of neuroleptic drug may be longer than anticholinergic, and dystonic reaction may otherwise come back again in a few hours.

- Serotonin Syndrome may at times be difficult to distinguish from NMS. Shivering, diarrhea (GI symptoms), tremor, hyperreflexia, and myoclonus tend to point more toward Serotonin Syndrome. Rigidity and very high creatine phosphokinase (CPK) levels tend to point more toward NMS.
- SSRI Discontinuation Syndrome mnemonic:
AMINES:
A → Adrenergic excess symptoms
M → Mood fluctuations
IN → Intestinal flu-like illness
E → Extrapyramidal symptoms
S → Sleep disturbances
- In order to distinguish SSRI Discontinuation Syndrome from recurrence of Major Depressive Episode, consider the following when reinstituting antidepressant:
If relief is in hours—think SSRI Discontinuation Syndrome.
If relief takes several days to weeks—think recurrence of Major Depressive Episode.

Chapter Self-Test Questions

Circle the correct answer. After you have responded to the questions, check your answers in Appendix A.

1. Self-destructive acts should:

a. *Always* be taken seriously.

b. *Frequently* be taken seriously.

c. *Never* be taken seriously.

d. *Sometimes* be taken seriously.

2. Suicide attempters and deaths by suicide are different, if overlapping, populations. Rates of suicide attempts are high among what age and gender, contrasting with demographic profile of suicide deaths.

a. Young females

b. Young males

c. Older females

d. Older males

3. Rates for death by suicide in patients with Personality Disorder alone may be less than those with Personality Disorder and comorbid:

    a. enduring pattern of inner experience and behavior that deviates markedly from the expectations of the individual's culture

    b. Chronic interpersonal difficulties

    c. Other Axis II pathology

    d. Severe Axis I pathology

4. Adolescent suicide rates are:

    a. Falling.

    b. Falling gradually.

    c. Rising.

    d. Staying the same.

5. In the United States, what race and gender are associated with the highest suicide rate?

    a. Black females

    b. Black males

    c. White females

    d. White males

 See the testbank CD for more self-test questions.

COGNITIVE AND SECONDARY ("ORGANIC") MENTAL DISORDERS

Michael R. Privitera, MD, MS and Jeffrey M. Lyness, MD

I. Overview [VI.1]

A. DSM-IV-TR adopted phrase "cognitive disorders and secondary syndromes"

B. "Organic": term often used clinically for secondary syndromes.

C. "Organic" in quotes because brain dysfunction (however subtle or poorly understood) *must* be a concomitant, although not necessarily a cause, of *all* psychiatric illness

D. *"Organic" mental disorder:* one or several known or presumed physical illnesses directly affecting brain function—leads to altered behavioral and symptomatic phenomena

E. *Cognitive symptoms:* pertain to attention, consciousness, language, speech, memory, and orientation in space

F. A psychiatric syndrome may be first or only manifestation of new medical or neurological process

G. Therefore, think "differential diagnosis" when evaluating psychiatric presentations

II. Etiologies [XVIII.7]

A. Intrinsic central nervous system (CNS) diseases

> It should make sense that disorders that are intrinsic CNS diseases may lead to psychiatric symptoms, because by definition they directly affect brain function.

1. Congenital defects
2. Toxins (e.g., lead)
3. Tumors (primary CNS or metastases to brain)
4. Cerebrovascular disorders (e.g., infarct, hemorrhage, vasculitis)
5. Infection (e.g., meningitis, encephalitis, human immunodeficiency virus [HIV], neurosyphilis)
6. Demyelination
7. Degeneration (e.g., Alzheimer's disease, Parkinson's disease)
8. Hydrocephalus (e.g., obstructive, normal pressure hydrocephalus)
9. Seizures (including auras and postictal and interictal states)

B. Systemic diseases

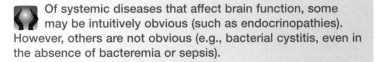 Of systemic diseases that affect brain function, some may be intuitively obvious (such as endocrinopathies). However, others are not obvious (e.g., bacterial cystitis, even in the absence of bacteremia or sepsis).

1. Infection (from isolated abscess or cystitis to full-blown sepsis)
2. Cardiovascular/hematological disorders (e.g., congestive heart failure, low cardiac output states, anemia, hyperviscosity states)
3. Metabolic disorders (e.g., hypoxemia, electrolyte disturbances, renal or hepatic failure, porphyria, burn-related disturbances, diabetes mellitus)
4. Endocrine disorders (e.g., of thyroid, adrenal cortex, medulla, pancreas, or sex hormones)
5. Nutritional deficiencies (e.g., vitamin B_{12}, thiamine, niacin)
6. Cancer

C. Drugs
1. Recreational and medicinal preparations can cause psychiatric syndromes by either *intoxication* or *withdrawal*
   a. *Intoxication:* in this context means having drug in one's system (even if in "therapeutic range")

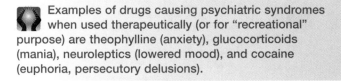 Examples of drugs causing psychiatric syndromes when used therapeutically (or for "recreational" purpose) are theophylline (anxiety), glucocorticoids (mania), neuroleptics (lowered mood), and cocaine (euphoria, persecutory delusions).

b. *Withdrawal:* refers to any state of reducing or eliminating drug from one's system

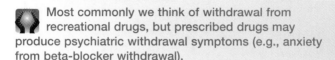 Most commonly we think of withdrawal from recreational drugs, but prescribed drugs may produce psychiatric withdrawal symptoms (e.g., anxiety from beta-blocker withdrawal).

2. Common offending drugs to keep in mind
    a. Drugs of recreational use, abuse, and dependence
    b. Psychotropics
    c. Anticholinergics
    d. Steroids (glucocorticoids and sex steroids)
    e. Histamine blockers
    f. Many antiarrhythmics (e.g., digoxin, lidocaine)
    g. Beta-adrenergic blockers

III. Phenomenological Types of Organic Mental Disorders
   A. Secondary syndromes
    1. Symptomatically resemble their idiopathic counterparts, although have an identifiable specific "organic" etiology
    2. DSM-IV-TR phrasing: _____ (psychiatric syndrome) Due to _____ (etiology)
    3. Named according to characteristic feature
        a. Psychotic Disorder Due to _____ (specify delusions, hallucinations)
        b. Anxiety Disorder Due to _____
        c. Delusional Disorder Due to _____
        d. Mood Disorder Due to _____ (specify depressed, manic, etc.)
        e. Personality Change Due to _____
        f. Sleep Disorder Due to _____
        g. Sexual Disorder Due to _____
   B. Cognitive disorders
    1. By virtue of prominent cognitive deficits, are usually distinguishable from idiopathic psychiatric disorders
        a. Those with *global* cognitive deficits (more than one realm of cognition is affected)
            i. Delirium
            ii. Dementia

b. *Mono*deficit disorders

    i. Amnestic Disorder: deficit of impaired memory only

  2. In all cases, etiology should be specified when known (e.g., Dementia Due to Cerebrovascular Disease)

IV. Delirium

A. Overview

  1. Definition: transient fluctuating global cognitive dysfunction

  2. Importance (VI 4–5, XVIII 5–6)

    a. Has enormously *high prevalence* in medically ill populations, such as those found on medical/surgical floors

    b. Associated with increased rates of *morbidity* and *mortality* for short term (e.g., in hospital) and long term

    c. May be first or most prominent manifestation of change in patient's physical (medical) status

  3. Should be *regarded as medical emergency until proved otherwise* (though for many patients, does have nonemergent etiology)

  4. Despite importance, delirium frequently missed or misdiagnosed. Possible reasons:

    a. *Semantic muddle:* varied terms tend to hamper clinicians from thinking of delirium as a common core psychiatric syndrome (e.g., encephalopathy, acute organic brain syndrome)

    b. *Often is multifactorial* (e.g., hematocrit of 32, sodium of 131, mild congestive heart failure, and arterial O_2 saturation of 87%): individually these factors may not cause delirium, but together they may.

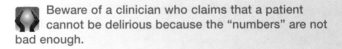 Beware of a clinician who claims that a patient cannot be delirious because the "numbers" are not bad enough.

    c. Despite clinical syndrome of delirium, sometimes there is no evident cause

Similarly, beware of clinicians who claim the patient "cannot have delirium" because clinicians "cannot find a cause." If the patient has the clinical syndrome, then the patient has delirium. It is your job to find out why. You may not find out the cause, but ignorance of the etiology should not make you pretend the syndrome is not present.

d. Delirium can be quite varied in clinical manifestations ("protean" accurately describes delirium)
  i. Core features define syndrome
  ii. Multiple associated symptoms may be more prominent than core symptoms
B. Core features of delirium
  1. Acute onset (typically hours to days rather than weeks to months)
  2. Transient (usually lasts days to several weeks, usually ending in complete resolution or death)
  3. Fluctuating ("waxing and waning") course (patients may look different one moment to next; from lucidity to disorientation and vice versa)

 Wide variation in lucidity is an excellent tip-off to delirium.

  4. Altered level of consciousness (key feature, as lethargy and stupor are not part of most idiopathic psychiatric disorders)
  5. Impaired attention (may be evident as distractibility or perseveration during conversation, not just on formal testing)
  6. Disorientation (severe disorientation to place or time is unusual in idiopathic psychiatric disorders)
  7. Other cognitive impairment (anything or everything)
    a. Memory
    b. Language
    c. Praxis
    d. Visual-spatial
  8. Disorganized thinking (e.g., loosening of associations)
C. Other common associated features
  1. Mood disturbance (sad, euphoric, anxious, irritable)
  2. Psychosis (delusions, hallucinations, thought process derailments)
  3. Psychomotor changes (agitation, slowing)
  4. Disturbed sleep-wake cycle (from mild insomnia or hypersomnia to total loss of 24-hour rhythms)
  5. Nonlateralizing neurological findings (subtle tremor, dysarthria, and gait ataxia)

PART

Correct diagnosis has treatment implications in distinguishing major depression from hypoactive delirium, as giving antidepressants to a delirious patient may worsen the delirium.

D. Assessment [XVIII 8]
1. Routine
    a. Symptom history: time course, fluctuations, cognitive deficits characteristic of core syndrome
    b. Thorough medical history (including detailed medication and drug history): will usually give clues to most likely causes of delirium
    c. Physical examination: as comprehensive as clinical state allows, looking for proceses that may contribute to delirium
    d. Neurological examination: particularly important to search for focal or specific CNS processes and nonfocal stigmata (i.e., tremor, dysarthria, gait ataxia) that accompany drug-induced or metabolic delirium
    e. Mental status examination: must include detailed cognitive assessment
2. Following are ordered per clinical picture
    a. Laboratory evaluations: if no clues as to etiology of delirium up to this point, proceed to laboratory evaluations immediately
        i. First level: complete blood count (CBC), electrolyte levels, glucose, blood urea nitrogen (BUN), creatinine, liver enzymes, arterial partial pressure of oxygen (Pao_2) or oximetry saturation, urinalysis and toxicology screen
        ii. Next level: thyroid-stimulating hormone (TSH), serum thyroxine (T_4), vitamin B_{12}, folate, rapid plama reagin (RPR), and consderation of human immunodeficiency virus (HIV) testing, serum ammonia, and serum albumin
        iii. Consider the example of a young, previously healthy patient with clear-cut delirium after overdose of diazepam (Valium); no abnormalities on physical examination outside of dysarthria and gait unsteadiness; you may check a few or no laboratories as delirium workup (although you may want to order tests as part of workup for the overdose itself)

b. Other testing

   i. First level: electrocardiogram (ECG), chest x-ray

  ii. Next level: neuroimaging study with computed tomography (CT) scan as easiest and most available means, followed by lumbar puncture (LP), possibly electroencephalogram (EEG)—(shows generalized slowing in most deliria and characteristic fast-wave pattern in alcohol withdrawal delirium)

> On rare occasions EEG might help clarify diagnosis of delirium in cases of atonic (i.e., no gross motor activity) status epilepticus or in differential diagnosis of psychosis of delirium versus idiopathic psychiatric disorder.

E. Treatment of Delirium

  1. Far and away most important: treat underlying condition as much as possible

  2. Avoid all CNS-active drugs as much as you can—especially avoid benzodiazepines, which are notorious for making delirium worse

  3. Consider change of suspected-but-needed therapeutic medication to one potentially less CNS-toxic

  4. If life-threatening agitation (e.g., hitting caregivers, pulling out needed intravenous (IV) lines) and nonpharmacological approaches, such as calm, quiet milieu or restraints, do not work sufficently, low doses of high-potency first-generation antipsychotic drugs, such as haloperidol (PO or IV), or low doses of second-generation antipsychotic drugs risperidone, olanzapine, aripiprazole, ziprasidone, or quetiapine may reduce agitation and psychosis without worsening delirium.

> Remember that when a patient is delirious, a previously normally functioning person may quickly become paranoid and believe he is defending his life. Delirium is associated with a great number of staff injuries as a result of the above.

V. Dementia

A. Overview **VI 6–8**

1. Definition: a syndrome of global cognitive impairment, including memory disturbance, and at least one other cognitive realm; there are many possible causes (Box 8.1).

2. Onset: after childhood, which distinguishes it from Mental Retardation

3. Most commonly, a chronic progressive disease affecting elderly

4. Younger patients are not entirely free from risk (e.g., Dementia Due to Traumatic Brain Injury, HIV disease)

5. Some dementia syndromes improve or resolve: therefore, do not give up too soon on differential diagnosis or assume prognosis is hopeless

6. Many people (especially in older age groups) have at least some amount of cognitive impairment, yet do not have dementia

7. Severity of impairments: cognitive deficits must interfere with patient's functional level to count as dementia

    a. Knowledge of person's previous functional level is often crucial; for example:

> Highly educated intelligent person with mild dementing disorder may still be more intelligent and intellectually functional than much of general population, yet functional decline from baseline justifies diagnosis of dementia.

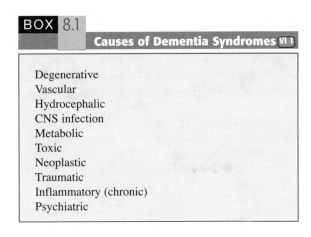

BOX 8.1

Causes of Dementia Syndromes **VI 1**

Degenerative
Vascular
Hydrocephalic
CNS infection
Metabolic
Toxic
Neoplastic
Traumatic
Inflammatory (chronic)
Psychiatric

8. Associated psychiatric symptoms with Dementia
   a. Personality change (an exaggeration of premorbid traits or onset of new traits)
   b. Mood disturbance (depression, euphoria, anxiety, irritability)
   c. Psychosis (in Dr. Alzheimer's original case report, persecutory delusions were the patient's main presenting symptom)
   d. Sleep disturbance
   e. Other "nonspecific" behavioral disturbances (e.g., yelling, aggessivity, wandering)
B. Assessment VI 8
   1. Assessment similar in broad outline to that of delirium
   2. Careful history, physical (including neurological) examination, and mental status examination usually sufficient to make diagnosis and suggest likely etiology
   3. Most clinicians agree: in newly presenting dementia, check battery of blood and urine tests cited for delirium, and order ECG and chest x-ray
   4. Unlike delirium, clear-cut dementia syndrome in and of itself not a medical emergency
   5. To date, there are no laboratory findings pathognomonic for Alzheimer's disease (most common cause of dementia)
   6. Diagnosis of Alzheimer's disease, although usually accurate, must technically be considered "probable" until confirmed at autopsy
   7. Reasonable opinions differ as to usefulness and cost-effectiveness of routine neuroimaging studies
      a. Any features in workup that are atypical for Alzheimer's disease or that raise possibility of more specific neurological process should lead to appropriate neuroimaging scan (generally magnetic resonance imaging [MRI] or CT)
   8. Lumbar puncture and EEG not part of routine evaluation of dementia and should be reserved for cases in which specifically indicated
   9. Table 8.1 describes major subtypes of dementia.
C. Treatment of Dementia
   1. Treatment differs from delirium as most causes are not reversible.
   2. Risk factors for disease progression (e.g., hypertension, diabetes mellitus) should be managed aggressively.
   3. Comorbid conditions that may contribute partially to dementia should be treated aggressively.

TABLE 8.1	Major Subtypes of Dementia VI 6.8			
	Alzheimer's Disease	Vascular	Frontotemporal (Pick's is variant)	Dementia With Lewy's Bodies
Frequency (at autopsy)	50%–70%	13%–16%	Overall: 1%–5% If <65 years old: 12%–22%	15%–35%
Etiological factors	Extraneuronal: beta-amyloid Intraneuronal: destabilization of tau protein	Cortical: large cerebral vessel strokes Subcortical: small lacunar infarcts	Spherical intracytoplasmic inclusion bodies, hyperphosphorylated tau proteins (if Pick's)	Intracytoplasmic protein deposits (Lewy's bodies)
Usual onset	Most begin >65 years old	After vascular pathology	Usually 40–60 years old, range 20–80 years old	Usually older age
Typical symptoms	Usual cognitive impairments associated with dementia syndrome	Cortical: depends on location Subcortical: often frontal lobe impairments	Early behavioral and language disturbance, often before other cognitive impairments Compulsive, bizarre delusions, hypersexual, apathy, unusual oral habits, inappropriate social conduct, frontal lobe symptoms	Fluctuating cognitive symptoms, visual hallucinations, parkinsonism, falls, syncope

| **Treatment issues** | Acetylcholinesterase inhibitors
NMDA antagonist | ↓ Risk factors for stroke
Acetylcholinesterase inhibitors | Not well established | Avoid neuroleptics; very sensitive to neuroleptics → can cause acute impairment as delirium symptoms.*
Use acetylcholinesterase inhibitors, which may improve cognitive, apathy, anxiety, delusions, and hallucinations |

*Parkinson's Disease with Dementia does not have the same cognitive deterioration with neuroleptic drugs but has potential to get worse in extrapyramidal symptoms (depending on choice of antipsychotic agent).

    a. Often this involves simplification of medication regimens and, particularly, minimizing use of CNS medications that exacerbate cognitive symptoms

  4. Even when nothing further can be done to treat the cause of dementia, much can be offered to patients and their families.

    a. Mood, psychotic, or other behavioral symptoms often respond well to pharmacological therapy, nonpharmacological interventions such as behavioral therapies, or both.

    b. Supportive psychotherapies with patient (in earlier phases of illness) and with families are essential to help educate, support, and guide them through complex and difficult decisions and tasks associated with such devastating chronic illnesses.

    c. Often crucial are education and guidance regarding use of appropriate agencies and community resources.

      i. Home health care, residential facilities

      ii. Attention to financial and legal issues raised by potential loss of competency of patients to care for or make decisions for themselves

VI. Distinguishing Delirium and Dementia (VI 3 and XVIII 5)

  A. Delirium and dementia are both disorders of global cognitive impairment but have very different implications for:

    1. Prognosis.

    2. Extent of urgency and depth of evaluation.

    3. Treatment.

  B. Delirium and dementia often coexist.

    1. Preexisting dementia is risk factor for becoming delirious with new physiological insult.

    2. Some acutely delirious patients will be found to have underlying dementia when delirium clears.

  C. Table 8.2 describes the differential diagnosis of delirium and dementia.

MENTOR TIPS DIGEST

• It should make sense that disorders that are intrinsic CNS diseases may lead to psychiatric symptoms, because by definition they directly affect brain function.

TABLE 8.2	Differential Diagnosis of Delirium and Dementia* VI 2–3	
	Delirium	Dementia
Onset	Acute, rapid (does not rule out Dementia from some causes; e.g., traumatic brain injury)	Gradual and insidious (over months or years)
Course	Fluctuating (waxing and waning)	Usually progressive
Primary Cognitive Deficits	Attention, memory, level of consciousness, orientation	Memory (without inattention), language, visual-spatial skills, praxis
Hallucinations	Usually visual; can also be auditory, gustatory, olfactory, tactile	Visual or auditory
Delusions	Usually persecutory but fleeting and fragmented	Usually paranoid, often fixed
Reversibility	Usual	Not usual

*These are guidelines as a starting point (but no broad postulates suffice for all situations).

- Of systemic diseases that effect brain function, some may be intuitively obvious (such as endocrinopathies). However, others are not obvious (e.g., bacterial cystitis, in the absence of bacteremia or sepsis).
- Examples of drugs causing psychiatric syndromes even used therapeutically (or for 'recreational' purpose) are theophylline (anxiety), glucocorticoids (mania), neuroleptics (lowered mood), and cocaine (persecutory delusions).

- Most commonly we think of withdrawal from recreational drugs, but prescribed drugs may produce psychiatric withdrawal symptoms (e.g., anxiety from beta-blocker withdrawal).
- Beware of a clinician who claims that a patient cannot be delirious because the "numbers" are not bad enough.
- Similarly, beware of clinicians who claim the patient "cannot have delirium" because clinicians "cannot find a cause." If the patient has the clinical syndrome, then the patient has delirium. It is your job to find out why. You may not find out the cause, but ignorance of the etiology should not make you pretend the syndrome is not present.
- Wide variation in lucidity is an excellent tip-off to delirium.
- Correct diagnosis has treatment implications in distinguishing major depression from hypoactive delirium, as giving antidepressants to a delirious patient may worsen the delirium.
- On rare occasions EEG might help clarify diagnosis of delirium in such cases of atonic (i.e., no gross motor activity) status epilepticus or in differential diagnosis of psychosis of delirium versus idiopathic psychiatric disorder.
- Remember that when a patient is delirious, a previously normal functioning person may quickly become paranoid and believe that they are defending their life. Delirium is associated with a great number of staff injuries as a result of the above.
- Highly educated intelligent person with mild dementing disorder, may still be more intelligent and intellectually functional than much of general population, yet functional decline from baseline qualifies him to be considered demented.

Resources

Agronin ME: Dementia. Philadelphia, Lippincott Williams & Wilkins, 2004.
Levenson JL (ed): Textbook of Psychosomatic Medicine. Washington DC, American Psychiatric Publishing Inc, 2005.

Chapter Self-Test Questions

Circle the correct answer. After you have responded to the questions, check your answers in Appendix A.

1. Secondary mental disorders are those disorders with psychiatric symptoms attributable to a disorder of brain dysfunction. Which of the following is a clinical term often used to refer to such secondary syndromes?

   a. Objective

   b. Organelle

   c. Organic

   d. Orphan

2. The mental functions of attention, consciousness, language, speech, memory, and visuospatial skills are grouped together and pertain to one domain of symptom categories. This domain is referred to by which of the following terms?

   a. Cognitive

   b. Motor

   c. Psychotic

   d. Somatoform

3. Secondary psychiatric disorders are syndromes that are thought to be attributable to a discernible brain dysfunction. Which of the following is currently considered a possible "organic" etiology?

   a. Chemical compounds containing carbon

   b. Foods grown with only natural fertilizers

   c. Intrinsic CNS disease

   d. Low levels of serotonin

4. An example of a drug that is well known to cause a psychiatric syndrome of anxiety even when used therapeutically is:

   a. Buspirone.

   b. Lorazepam.

   c. Olanzapine.

   d. Theophylline.

5. Which of the following drug classes is known to cause a syndrome of mania, even at therapeutic doses?

   a. Beta-adrenergic blockers

   b. Calcium channel blockers

   c. Glucocorticoids

   d. Mood stabilizers

See the testbank CD for more self-test questions.

9
CHAPTER

MOOD DISORDERS

Michael R. Privitera, MD, MS, and Jeffrey M. Lyness, MD

I. Introduction

A. Mood Disorders are mental disorders in which disturbances of emotion predominate.

B. Lifetime prevalence for any mood disorder: ~20% for both sexes. (X 2)

C. Mood Disorders are subdivided: Depressive Disorders, Bipolar Disorders, and Other Mood Disorders.

II. Clinical Features Disorders are made up of episodes; specifiers describe current episode or clinical course of episodes

A. Episodes: building blocks of disorders; episodes are Major Depressive, Manic, Mixed, or Hypomanic; pattern of presentation during patient lifetime defines diagnosis (dx).

> ⚡ **DIAGNOSTIC TIP:** Clinically, the "great divide" is the distinction between unipolar and bipolar illnesses. Both manifest episodes of depression, but bipolar illnesses are also characterized by episodes of mania or hypomania.

1. Major Depressive Episode (MDE): 2-week or longer period of five or more of the following symptoms, present most of the day nearly every day, at least one being either depressed mood or loss of interest or pleasure (anhedonia): (X 4)
   a. Sleep: insomnia or hypersomnia
   b. Interest: loss of interest or pleasure, or depressed mood
   c. Guilt: thoughts of guilt or worthlessness
   d. Energy: loss of energy; fatigue
   e. Concentration: diminished ability to concentrate or make decisions

f. Appetite: changes in appetite or weight
g. Psychomotor: psychomotor retardation or agitation
h. Suicide: suicidal thoughts, preoccupation with death

 DIAGNOSTIC TIP: SIG: E CAPS ("prescribe energy capsules") is a useful mnemonic for remembering the symptoms of a Major Depressive Episode: S = Sleep, I = Interest, G = Guilt, E = Energy, C = Concentration, A = Appetite, P = Psychomotor, S = Suicide.

DIAGNOSTIC TIP: Remember to always ask about a past history of hypomanic/manic symptoms to help rule out bipolar depression.

DIAGNOSTIC TIP: Because *depressed mood* or *anhedonia* needs to be present in a Major Depressive Episode, asking about both of these is a very useful screening technique. Ask about the rest of the symptoms of depression if one or both are positive.

 WORKUP TIP:
Essential: physical exam, thyroid-stimulating hormone (TSH), urinalysis
If difficult diagnosis: add chemical dependency screen, metabolic screening, consider electrocardiogram (ECG), chest x-ray (CXR), neuroimaging
If treatment (tx)-resistant: neuroimaging, electroencephalogram (EEG) with T_1/T_2 montages

2. *Manic episode:* 1 week or longer period (any duration if hospitalization is necessary) of elevated (euphoric), expansive, or irritable mood *plus* three of the following symptoms (four if only irritable) (IX 4):
   a. Distractibility
   b. Decreased need for sleep (quite different from anguished insomnia of depression)
   c. Grandiosity or inflated self-esteem
   d. Flight of ideas or racing thoughts
   e. Psychomotor agitation (e.g., pacing, fidgeting, physical aggressivity) or increase in goal-directed activity

f. Excessive involvement in pleasurable activities (e.g., spending sprees, hypersexuality, foolish business deals, incessant letter writing, telephone calling)

g. Pressured speech (and increased in amount [logorrhea], talkativeness, often loud)

> **DIAGNOSTIC TIP:** A useful mnemonic for a manic episode is (mood = elated, expansive, or irritable) plus DIGFAST: D = Distractibility, I = Insomnia, G = Grandiosity, F = Flight of ideas, A = Activity, Agitation & Ambitiousness, S = Sex & Spending, T = Talkative.

> **WORKUP TIP:**
> *Essential:* physical exam, TSH, chemical dependency screen
> *Difficult dx or tx-resistant cases:* metabolic screening, urinalysis, consider ECG, chest x-ray (CXR), neuroimaging.

3. *Mixed episode:* combination of criteria for *both* manic and major depressive episodes (except both are for at least 1 week) and causing marked impairment

> **DIAGNOSTIC TIP:** You may hear the clinical term *dysphoric mania*, which is another label for what DSM-IV calls Bipolar Disorder, Mixed.

4. *Hypomanic episode:* minimum of 4-day period of elevated, expansive, or irritable mood with three or more (four if mood is only irritable) manic symptoms, except not severe enough to cause marked impairment socially or occupationally, without psychosis, but sufficient to be uncharacteristic of the person when not symptomatic and are observable by others

> **DIAGNOSTIC TIP:** Hypomania is essentially mania without drawbacks, e.g., without substantial impairment in social or occupational functioning.

B. Specifiers
  1. Current or most recent episode :
    a. *Severity:* mild, moderate, or severe

    b. *Psychotic:* hallucinations, delusions, or derailments of thought process

    c. *Remission:* partial or full

    d. *Chronic:* major depressive episode for ≥2 years

    e. *Catatonic:* motor immobility, excessive motor activity, extreme negativism, posturing, echolalia, or echopraxia

    f. *Melancholic:* anhedonia, lack of reactivity to pleasant circumstances, distinct quality of mood (different than loss of a loved one), diurnal variation (mornings worse), early morning awakening, psychomotor retardation or agitation, anorexia, weight loss, and severe guilt

    g. *Atypical:* mood reactivity, with two or more of: weight gain/increased appetite, hypersomnia and leaden paralysis—heavy feeling in arms or legs, longstanding interpersonal rejection sensitivity; affects patient socially or occupationally

    h. *Postpartum onset:* onset within 4 months postpartum

2. Pattern of episodes (Fig. 9.1)

    a. *Full interepisode recovery:* full remission between episodes

    b. *Seasonal pattern:* regular temporal relationship of onset of major depressive episode—over 2 years and particular time of the year—not obviously related to seasonally occurring psychosocial stressor, full remissions or episode switches at characteristic times of the year, and seasonal → nonseasonal episodes over lifetime

    c. *Rapid cycling:* four or more mood episodes in previous 12-month period

C. Disorders

  1. Depressive disorders:

    a. Overview

 Although DSM-IV-TR simply lists symptoms, it is useful clinically to consider them in clusters of symptom types:

     i. *Mood:* dysphoria (obviously), but also possible are nonreactivity of mood, anxiety, irritability

     ii. *Ideational/psychological:* thoughts of worthlessness, guilt, helplessness, hopelessness, decreased interests, anhedonia, decreased subjective ability to concentrate, suicidal

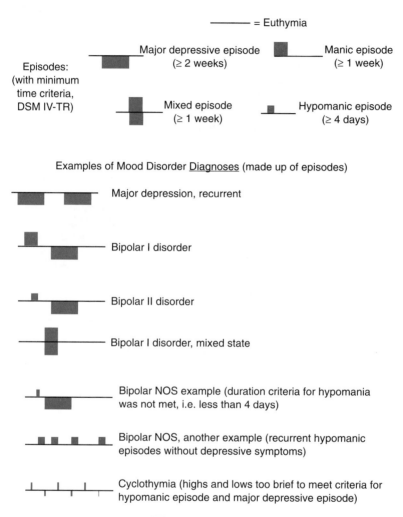

FIGURE 9.1 **Mood diagrams.**

thoughts or behavior, ruminative thinking (tendency to dwell on the same depressive theme; often somatic/nihilistic themes predominate)

iii. *Neurovegetative:* sleep change (insomnia or hypersomnia), appetite and weight changes (up or down), anergia, decreased libido, psychomotor change (agitation and/or retardation), diurnal variation (most commonly mornings worse)

iv. *Neuropsychological:* decreased performance on cognitive testing, usually related to poor effort and attention; occasionally (especially in the elderly) more profound impairment but generally distinguishable from that seen in degenerative dementia such as Alzheimer's disease

v. *Functional:* social withdrawal, impaired performance at work, school, or other tasks: in severe cases, hygiene or other basic personal tasks may be affected

WORKUP TIP: The word "depression" is regrettably nonspecific: it can refer to *mood state* (either normal or in a psychopathological state), *clinical syndrome* (e.g., major depressive syndrome due to hypothyroidism), or a *specific disorder*. Think differential diagnosis when evaluating depressive symptoms.

DIAGNOSTIC TIP: Remember to look for the *criteria* for each disorder. Do not be distracted (diagnostically) by whether there was a precipitating stressor associated with onset of the mood symptoms; e.g.:
Major depressive episode may occur with or without a precipitant.
Adjustment disorder and Bereavement (not pathological) both have a precipitant, but the symptom criteria are what will help you distinguish among these conditions.

DIAGNOSTIC TIP: Delusions are the most common psychotic symptom in unipolar depression with psychotic features; when present, often mood-congruent. Hallucinations are most commonly auditory.

b. Major Depressive Disorder
   i. Definition: Idiopathic condition having one or more Major Depressive Episodes
   ii. Onset: peak in late 20s, but can be childhood to late life

   iii. Epidemiology ⓍⓏ
     (1) Most common mood disorder
     (2) Point prevalence: 8%–10% females, 3%–5% males
     (3) Lifetime prevalence: 20%–25% females, 8%–13% males
     (4) Prevalence increasing with younger age cohorts
     (5) Course: highly recurrent, with 5-year recurrence rate
       (A) 50% after first episode
       (B) 70% after second episode
       (C) 90% after third episode
   iv. Presentation
     (1) Most present first to primary care
     (2) Physical as well as psychological symptoms
     (3) Diagnosis often missed if not asked about
   v. Pathogeneses Ⓧ❶
     (1) Heterogeneous pathogeneses, although substantial similarity in clinical presentation
     (2) Pathogenetic mechanisms span biopsychosocial gamut: genetic and neurobiological, variety of psychological (including psychodynamic and cognitive) and psychosocial (e.g., family and cultural) theories
  c. Dysthymic Disorder
    i. Definition: chronic disorder (at least 2 years), of lesser degree and fewer (must include three) symptoms in number than Major Depression, but still can be very disabling
    ii. Onset: subdivided into early onset (<21 years) and late onset (≥21 years)
   iii. Epidemiology Ⓧ❷
     (1) Point prevalence: 5%
     (2) Lifetime prevalence: 6.4% (8% female, 5% male)
     (3) Course: chronic by definition
   iv. Presentation
     (1) Because chronic, often misdiagnosed as part of patient's personality or missed
     (2) May respond to pharmacotherapy and other therapies, but because chronic, prognosis may be guarded
  d. Depressive Disorder Not Otherwise Specified (NOS)
    i. Definition: any depressive disorder not meeting criteria for Major Depressive Disorder, Dysthymic Disorder, or any Adjustment Disorder

2. Bipolar Disorders:

> It is clinically useful to cluster psychopathological symptoms in Bipolar Disorders in groups that are associated with three distinct neurobiological mechanisms that are orthogonal axes to each other (Fig. 9.2). This more pathophysiological approach will allow better assessment of worsening or improvement along these axes, and treatment interventions may be more specifically and rationally selected.

  a. Central Pleasure Reward mechanisms:
    i. Depression: inhibition of pleasure
    ii. Mania: disinhibition of pleasure
  b. Central Pain Disturbance:
    i. Depression: disinhibition of pain
    ii. Mania: inhibition of pain
  c. Psychomotor Regulation
    i. Depression: deceleration
    ii. Mania: acceleration

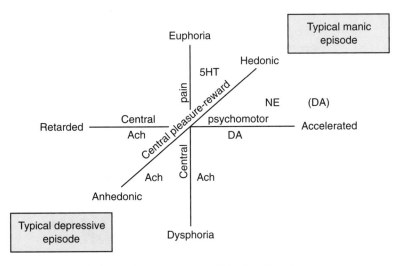

FIGURE 9.2 Psychobiologic parameters of bipolar disorder. (Courtesy of B. J. Carroll, MD, PhD, personal communication.)

DIAGNOSTIC TIP: Episodes of depression in bipolar disorder often resemble those in unipolar disorder but are more likely to demonstrate reversed neurovegetative signs (hypersomnia, hyperphagia, weight gain).

 Psychosis (including prominent hallucinations or thought process disturbance; seen more rarely in unipolar depression) may be present.

 Poor response to nonsomatic therapies alone is typical.

d. Overview
  i. Idiopathic conditions
  ii. Characterized by recurrent episodes of manic/hypomanic plus major depressive symptoms or episodes; a rare form exists that never has depressive episodes (called "unipolar mania")
  iii. Usually good interepisode functioning
  iv. Causes are probably not as heterogeneous as those of unipolar depressions
  v. Neurobiological factors, including genetics, probably predominant in most or all cases
  vi. Psychological and social factors often related to timing and triggering of acute episodes (especially situations that lead to poor sleep) and affect long-term outcome, including treatment compliance and alliance with caregivers
  vii. More time usually spent in depressive than manic episodes
  viii. Each phase can have devastating and painful consequences
e. Bipolar I Disorder

 DIAGNOSTIC TIP: Compare Schizoaffective Disorder Bipolar Type that has bipolar mood episodes plus at least a 2-week period of *psychosis that is independent of mood episodes.*

  i. Definition
    (1) One or more full manic episodes

(2) Usually has major depressive episodes

(3) May also have hypomanic or mixed episodes

ii. Onset: most commonly young adulthood, can be adolescence, midlife, or (rarely) late life

iii. Epidemiology 🆇❷

    (1) Equal gender distribution

    (2) Point prevalence 0.5%–1%

    (3) Lifetime prevalence as high as 1.6%

    (4) Course: recurrence is the rule; usually but not always returns to healthy baseline between episodes

f. Bipolar II Disorder

  i. Definition

    (1) One or more hypomanic episodes

    (2) No full-fledged manic episodes

  ii. Epidemiology 🆇❷

    (1) Lifetime prevalence 0.5%

    (2) Generally one or more major depressive episodes

    (3) Course: most patients improve between episodes

  iii. Pathogeneses: genetics appear distinct from unipolar depression and Bipolar I

g. Cyclothymic Disorder

> **WORKUP TIP:** Cyclothymia may be hard to distinguish from affective instability of severe character pathology.

  i. Definition: periods of hypomanic or depressive symptoms not fulfilling criteria for hypomanic or major depressive episodes

  ii. Epidemiology: lifetime prevalence 0.4%–1% 🆇❷

h. Bipolar Disorder NOS

  i. Bipolar features but not meeting criteria for a specific Bipolar Disorder

3. Other mood disorders

a. Mood Disorder Due to a General Medical Condition

  i. Depressive, elated, or irritable mood symptoms or anhedonia causing significant distress or impairment

  ii. Symptoms physiologically due to a general medical condition

TABLE 9.1

Differential Diagnosis: Major Depression, Adjustment Disorder With Depressed Mood, and Bereavement IX 5

	Major Depression	Adjustment Disorder With Depressed Mood	Bereavement
Distinction	Illness	Probable illness	Normal, expected reaction to life situation
Symptoms	Multiple, moods, thoughts, bodily functions; can have: guilt about things other than actions taken/not taken by survivor, morbid preoccupation with worthlessness, marked psychomotor retardation, prolonged and marked functional impairment, hallucinations other than transiently of the deceased person	Few, nonvegetative (does not meet MDE criteria)	Essentially mood, sometimes insomnia, anorexia, anxiety
Duration	Persists	Onset within 3 months, duration ≤6 months	<2 months (generally)

(continued on page 128)

TABLE 9.1	Differential Diagnosis: Major Depression, Adjustment Disorder With Depressed Mood, and Bereavement IX 5 (continued)		
	Major Depression	Adjustment Disorder With Depressed Mood	Bereavement
Suicidal Potential	Suicidal ideation (SI) can occur, can result in suicide	Rarely with SI, but *can*	Usually no SI
Treatment	Specific medical/ psychiatric treatment; somatic treatment with or without psychotherapy as indicated	Good listener/support/t ime/brief symptomatic treatment (e.g., of insomnia, anorexia, anxiety) Consider antidepressants if stressor is ongoing and severe.	Good listener/ support/ time/brief symptomatic treatment

    iii. Not better accounted for by stress of having the medical condition
    iv. Not occurring exclusively during delirium
  b. Substance-Induced Mood Disorder
    i. Depressive, elated, or irritable mood symptoms or anhedonia causing significant distress or impairment
    ii. Symptoms judged to be due to substance intoxication or withdrawal
    iii. Symptoms are not better accounted for by non-substance-induced mood disorder
    iv. Not occurring exclusively during delirium
  c. Mood Disorder NOS

        i. Symptoms do not meet criteria for a specific mood disorder and difficult to categorize as either depressive disorder NOS or bipolar disorder NOS

  4. Other mood-related syndromes

    a. Syndromes that have depressive symptomatology often associated with recent life stressor (e.g., major life event, death of a loved one) need to be distinguished from major depressive episode (Table 9.1)

III. Differential Diagnosis

A. Depressive or manic symptoms

  1. Distinguish from delirium or dementia by ensuring there are not prominent cognitive deficits

  2. Distinguish from secondary mood disorder (due to general medical condition or substance-induced)

  3. Distinguish depressive from bipolar disorders by ensuring there is no previous history of hypomania or mania

  4. For depressive symptoms, if stressor as precipitant, distinguish from adjustment disorder, normal bereavement, or normal sadness

B. Irritability

  1. Seen in both depressive and bipolar disorders

  2. Distinguish by "company it keeps," i.e., what other symptoms are present?

C. Difficulties sustaining attention may be due to:

  1. Manic episode

  2. Hypomanic episode

  3. Delirium

  4. Attention-deficit hyperactivity disorder

IV. Treatment

A. Major Depressive Disorder

  1. Psychotherapy `IX 12`

    a. Best for:

      i. Mild to moderate depression

      ii. Obvious psychosocial stressors or interpersonal discord

      iii. Patients who cannot or will not accept or tolerate pharmacotherapy

    b. Demonstrated efficacy for:

      i. Cognitive psychotherapy

      ii. Interpersonal psychotherapy
      iii. Problem-solving therapy
   c. Often important roles for:
      i. Couples or family therapy
      ii. Group therapy
      iii. Other psychosocial interventions, e.g., day treatment program
2. Medications (IX 11)
   a. Best for:
      i. All types including severe depressions
      ii. Patients who cannot or will not accept or tolerate psychotherapy
   b. Antidepressant classes (Table 9.2)
   c. Other medications
      i. Adjuncts; e.g., benzodiazepines for short-term assistance with anxiety or insomnia
      ii. Augmentation: adding a different drug to enhance an antidepressant's efficacy; e.g., lithium, triiodothyronine, psychostimulant
3. Subtypes and treatment
   a. Melancholia: requires somatic therapies (antidepressants or electroconvulsive therapy [ECT]), will not do well with psychotherapy alone
   b. Psychotic: usually requires antidepressants plus antipsychotics, or ECT; some reports suggest that SSRIs alone work better than TCAs alone
   c. Seasonal: requires light therapy, antidepressants or both
4. Phases of treatment
   a. Three phases of treatment: acute, continuation, and maintenance
   b. Each phase has different implications in length of treatment and goals (Table 9.3)
   c. After first episode: treat through continuation phase, then consider whether to slowly taper over weeks and watch for recurrence
   d. After second episode: treat through continuation phase, and evaluate whether safe to consider coming off medications, based on severity, warning period of early prodrome, suicidality, psychosis, only "bread winner," etc.

TABLE 9.2
Antidepressant Classes and Examples

Class	Generic Name	Examples Trade Name(s)
TCA	amitriptyline	Elavil
	nortriptyline	Aventyl
	desipramine	Norpramin
	imipramine	Tofranil
SNRI	venlafaxine	Effexor (IR/XR)
	duloxetine	Cymbalta
	desvenlafaxine	Pristiq
SSRI	fluoxetine	Prozac
	sertraline	Zoloft
	paroxetine	Paxil
	citalopram	Celexa
	escitalopram	Lexapro
	fluvoxamine	Luvox
5HT-2 antagonist	trazodone	Desyrel
	nefazodone	Serzone
DNRI	bupropion	Wellbutrin (IR/SR/XL)
MAOI	tranylcypromine	Parnate
	phenelzine	Nardil
	selegeline skin patch	Emsam
NaSSA	mirtazapine	Remeron

TCA: tricyclic antidepressant
SNRI: serotonin norepinephrine reuptake inhibitor
SSRI: selective serotonin reuptake inhibitor
5HT-2 antagonist: serotonin-2 (postsynaptic) antagonist
DNRI: dopamine norepinephrine reuptake inhibitor
MAOI: monoamine oxidase inhibitor
NaSSA: norepinephrine and specific serotonin antidepressant

TABLE 9.3	**Treatment Phases of Major Depressive Disorder** (IX 11)		
	Acute Phase	**Continuation Phase**	**Maintenance Phase**
Goal	To get a **response**, then obtain full alleviation of symptoms, i.e., **remission**	After full **remission** has been achieved, keep the patient treated long enough to have fully treated the episode, i.e., to promote **recovery** and prevent **relapse**	After **recovery** for the episode, prevent further **recurrences**
Length	6–12 weeks	4–9 months	Taper off slowly or stay on medications indefinitely (based on number of previous episodes and their severity)
Treatment Issues	*Medications:* titrate doses, and/or use augmentation techniques to obtain **remission** *Psychotherapy:* frequency to obtain **remission**	*Medications:* dose that gets patient well (remission) keeps patient well. *Psychotherapy:* adjust frequency to keep wellness	*Medications:* thought to be same as continuation phase regarding doses, but less known; if choose to taper off antidepressant (e.g., after first episode), best to

Treatment Phases of Major Depressive Disorder IX-11 (continued)

Acute Phase	Continuation Phase	Maintenance Phase
		do *slowly* (over weeks) to enhance chances of successful taper *Psychotherapy:* less known, but thought to be similar to continuation phase

Recovery: remission long enough to treat the episode through continuation phase
Response: ≥50% reduction of symptoms
Remission: full resolution of symptoms
Relapse: return of symptoms after response or remission
Recurrence: return of symptoms after recovery, i.e., a new episode

    e. After third episode: remain on maintenance-phase medication indefinitely
B. Bipolar Disorder
    1. Primarily mood-stabilizing agents (e.g., lithium, divalproex, and some other anticonvulsants) to treat acute episodes and prevent recurrences
    2. In bipolar depression, avoid antidepressants alone, as they may precipitate a manic episode if prescribed in the absence of a mood stabilizer
    3. Antidepressants, antipsychotics, and anxiolytics are mostly reserved for acute exacerbations, but some patients require long-term use of these agents
    4. Lamotrigine useful in maintenance phase, especially helpful in bipolar depression; not ideal acute-phase medication due to slow titration
    5. Figure 9.3 shows typical bipolar treatment decisions

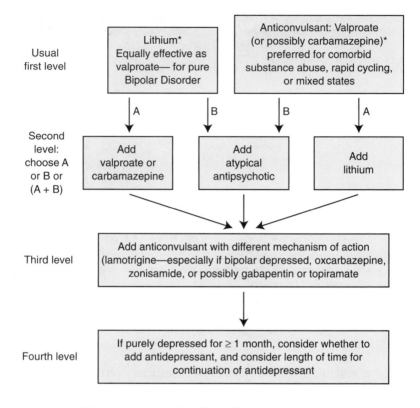

FIGURE 9.3 Bipolar treatment decisions. (These steps are provided as a guide only. Clinical situations that present themselves may necessitate a change in the order of these steps as indicated. For example, if mania were severe, one would start with an antipsychotic for the most rapid possible response.)

 MENTOR TIPS DIGEST

Mood Disorders Overall

- **DIAGNOSTIC TIP:** Clinically, the "great divide" is the distinction between unipolar and bipolar illnesses. Both manifest episodes of depression, but bipolar illnesses are also characterized by episodes of mania or hypomania.

Major Depressive Episode

- **DIAGNOSTIC TIP:** "SIG: E CAPS" ("prescribe energy capsules") is a useful mnemonic to remember the symptoms of a Major Depressive Episode: S = Sleep, I = Interest, G = Guilt, E = Energy, C = Concentration, A = Appetite, P = Psychomotor, S = Suicide.
- **DIAGNOSTIC TIP:** Remember to always ask about a past history of hypomanic/manic symptoms to help rule out bipolar depression.
- **DIAGNOSTIC TIP:** Because *depressed mood* or *anhedonia* needs to be present in a Major Depressive Episode, asking about both of these is a very useful screening technique. Ask about the rest of the symptoms of depression if one or both are positive.
- **WORKUP TIP:**
  Essential: physical exam, TSH, urinalysis.
  If difficult dx: add chemical dependency screen, metabolic screening, consider ECG, CXR, neuroimaging.
  If tx-resistant: neuroimaging, EEG with T_1/T_2 montages.

Manic Episode

- **DIAGNOSTIC TIP:** A useful mnemonic for a manic episode is (mood = elated, expansive, or irritable) plus DIGFAST: D = Distractibility, I = Insomnia, G = Grandiosity, F = Flight of ideas, A = Activity, Agitation & Ambitiousness, S = Sex & Spending, T = Talkative.
- **WORKUP TIP:**
  Essential: physical exam, TSH, chemical dependency screen.
  Difficult dx or tx-resistant cases: metabolic screening, urinalysis, consider ECG, CXR, neuroimaging.

Mixed Episode

- **DIAGNOSTIC TIP:** You may hear the clinical term *dysphoric mania*, which is another label for what DSM-IV calls Bipolar Disorder, Mixed.

Hypomanic Episode

- **DIAGNOSTIC TIP:** Hypomania is essentially mania without drawbacks, e.g., without substantial impairment in social or occupational functioning.

Depressive Disorders Although DSM-IV-TR simply lists symptoms, it is useful clinically to consider them in clusters of symptom types: Mood, Ideational/Psychological, Neurovegetative, Neuropsychological, and Functional.

- **WORKUP TIP:** The word "depression" is regrettably nonspecific. It can refer to *mood state* (either normal or in a psychopathological state), *clinical syndrome* (e.g., major depressive syndrome due to hypothyroidism), or a *specific disorder*. Think differential diagnosis when evaluating depressive symptoms.
- **DIAGNOSTIC TIP:** Remember to look for the *criteria* for each disorder. Do not be distracted (diagnostically) by whether there was a precipitating stressor associated with onset of the mood symptoms.
- **DIAGNOSTIC TIP:** Delusions are the most common psychotic symptom in unipolar depression with psychotic features; when present, often mood-congruent. Hallucinations are most commonly auditory.

Bipolar Disorders It is clinically useful to cluster psychopathological symptoms in bipolar disorders in groups that are associated with three distinct neurobiological mechanisms that are orthogonal axes to each other: Central Pleasure Reward mechanisms, Central Pain Disturbance, and Psychomotor Regulation.

- **DIAGNOSTIC TIP:** Episodes of depression in bipolar disorder often resemble those in unipolar disorder but are more likely to demonstrate reversed neurovegetative signs (hypersomnia, hyperphagia, weight gain). Psychosis (including prominent hallucinations or thought process disturbance, seen more rarely in unipolar depression) may be present. Poor response to nonsomatic therapies alone is typical.

Bipolar I Disorder

- **DIAGNOSTIC TIP:** Compare Schizoaffective Disorder Bipolar Type that has bipolar mood episodes plus at least a 2-week period of *psychosis that is independent of mood episodes.*

Cyclothymic Disorder

- **WORKUP TIP:** Cyclothymia may be hard to distinguish from affective instability of severe character pathology.

Resources

Carroll BJ: Psychopathology and Neurobiology of Manic-Depressive
   Disorders. In Carroll BJ and Barrett JE (eds): Psychopathology and the
   Brain. New York, Raven Press Ltd, 1991, pp 265-285.

Chapter Self-Test Questions

Circle the correct answer. After you have responded to the questions,
check your answers in Appendix A.

1. Given the prevalence of each mood disorder, when you are first evaluating a female patient for Major Depressive Episode, what is the estimated chance that this episode is part of a Bipolar Disorder?

   a. 1%

   b. 10%

   c. 50%

   d. 75%

2. When first evaluating a patient for Major Depressive Episode, why is it
   important to have asked about previous history of mania or hypomania
   before prescribing an antidepressant?

   a. Antidepressants alone in bipolar disorder may precipitate a
       hypomanic or manic episode, if mood stabilizers are not co-pre-
       scribed.

   b. Hypomanic history predicts a good response to antidepressants.

   c. The insurance company needs to know because antidepressants may
       be expensive compared with lithium.

   d. You can appear intelligent to your patient and his family.

3. For the diagnosis of a Major Depressive Episode, of the five criteria
   needed, at least one needs to be either depressed mood or:

   a. Anhedonia.

   b. Lack of energy.

   c. Lack of interest.

   d. Suicidal ideation.

4. Mixed episodes can be seen as part of the course of which of the following disorders?

a. Bipolar I disorder

b. Bipolar II disorder

c. Cyclothymic disorder

d. Dysthymic disorder

5. Which of the following does *not* meet the psychotic specifier criteria in a mood disorder?

a. Delusion

b. Hallucination

c. Loose association

d. Ruminative thinking

See the testbank CD for more self-test questions.

10
CHAPTER

PSYCHOTIC DISORDERS

**Michael R. Privitera, MD, MS, and
Jeffrey M. Lyness, MD**

I. Overview of Psychotic Symptoms

A. Psychotic symptoms come in three "flavors" `VIII 1`
  1. Hallucinations
  2. Delusions
  3. Thought-process disturbances (e.g., thought blocking, loose associations)
B. May be seen in a wide variety of psychiatric conditions, including dementia, delirium, mood disorders, and secondary ("organic") psychotic disorders, as well as the primary psychotic disorders discussed in this chapter `VIII 2`

> With psychotic *symptoms*, remember to think differential diagnosis.

C. Psychotic disorders are idiopathic conditions that manifest with psychotic symptoms, do not have prominent cognitive deficits (except as noted later), and with one exception (schizoaffective disorder) do not have prominent mood symptoms

II. Schizophrenia

A. Most common and important of psychotic disorders `VIII 4`
B. Prevalence and morbidity sufficient to make it a major public health problem
C. Schizophrenia does *not* mean "split personality" in sense of what is properly termed "multiple personality" (which was renamed Dissociative Identity Disorder in DSM-IV)
D. Schizophrenia: derived from Greek for *split mind*, referring to split between thoughts and affects sometimes seen in these patients

E. Hallmarks
   1. Must have periods of acute psychotic symptoms (delusions, hallucinations, disorganized speech, or grossly disorganized or catatonic behavior)
   2. May have *negative* symptoms
      a. Affective flattening
      b. Poverty of speech
      c. Avolition (lack of initiation of normal behaviors, such as grooming, dressing, seeking social interaction, pursuing goal-directed tasks)
   3. Episodes must include two or more of above symptoms (one symptom is enough if bizarre [non-plausible] delusions or specific types of auditory hallucinations)
   4. Cause social or occupational dysfunction
   5. Last longer than 6 months (including prodromal and residual symptoms)
      a. Prodromal and residual symptoms may include attenuated versions of psychotic symptoms or solely negative symptoms.
F. Course VIII 4
   1. Marked by periods of acute exacerbations
   2. Some patients might be largely symptom-free and quite functional between episodes
   3. Many patients are more chronically symptomatic
   4. Those patients with prominent and persistent negative symptoms tend to have more severe ongoing disability than those with solely "positive" (psychotic) symptoms
   5. "Positive" symptoms tend to respond better to acute treatments than do "negative" symptoms
   6. Different patterns of course exist
      a. Progressive illness
      b. Remain stable or improve symptomatically functionally or both over time
      c. Gradual or stepwise decline in functional ability
   7. Chronic and typically life-long illness
G. Theories of etiology and pathogenesis (run full biopsychosocial gamut)
   1. Prominent, current notions: emphasize role of neurobiology; combination of genetic, prenatal, perinatal, and early childhood–acquired factors VIII 3

2. Illness onset and subsequent acute clinical exacerbations can be related to stressful events and circumstances
H. Comorbidity
   1. Substantially affects treatment and prognosis
   2. Substance dependence: common comorbidity
      a. May add to patient's psychotic symptoms (e.g., Cocaine-Induced Psychotic Disorder)
      b. Such patients are referred to as "dual diagnosis" or MICA (mentally ill chemical abuser) patients
         i. Need treatment different from traditional psychiatric or substance-dependence treatment settings
         ii. Increasing array of outpatient and inpatient services is developing in many communities to serve specific needs of MICA patients
I. Syndromic differential diagnosis must confirm that phenomenology of psychosis not more consistent with another disorder
   1. Sole symptom of monothematic non-bizarre delusions is more consistent with delusional disorder
   2. Presence of prominent mood symptoms should raise possibility of schizoaffective disorder or primary mood disorder
   3. Prominent cognitive deficits should raise questions about underlying or even primary mental retardation or dementia (although may be difficult to assess in acutely disorganized patient)
      a. In residual stages of schizophrenia itself, subtle deficits may be found in areas such as frontal executive functions
   4. Secondary causes of psychosis must be sought (e.g., neuroimaging such as magnetic resonance imaging [MRI] in new-onset cases)

In differential diagnosis of psychotic symptoms, fundamentals remain, such as careful medical history, physical examination including neurological exam, and basic laboratory tests.

J. DSM-IV-TR describes subtypes of schizophrenia based on predominance of particular symptoms (e.g., paranoid, disorganized), although prognostic utility of these subtypes is limited
K. Treatment issues VIII 6
   1. Psychotropic drugs reduce frequency and severity of acute symptomatic exacerbations and improve quality of life for most people with schizophrenia.

a. Second-generation ("atypical") antipsychotics, such as quetiapine and risperidone, are the mainstay for many patients. Sometimes first-generation ("typical") antipsychotics, such as haloperidol, are used.

> *Metabolic* syndrome tends to be focus of general health maintenance of patients on atypical antipsychotics, and *tardive dyskinesia* or other *extrapyramidal symptoms* is the focus for patients on typical antipsychotics.

   b. Other drug classes play adjunctive roles, e.g., benzodiazepines in acute events, mood stabilizers.
2. Electroconvulsive therapy (ECT) may be used effectively for intractable acute psychosis or associated mood-related symptoms such as suicidal ideation.
3. Insight-oriented psychotherapy does not alter the basic psychopathogenesis of schizophrenia.
4. Psychotherapies of various types still play crucial roles in management of and dealing with this often chronic and debilitating disorder.
   a. Individual and group work usually focus on:
      i. Psychoeducation (including expectations regarding disease course and need for compliance with medications and follow-up treatment)
      ii. Support (helping minimize demoralization that may accompany profound disability)
5. Guidance with practical management of day-to-day affairs is provided by therapists and case-managers or by group settings including social programs for patients with similar needs.
6. Families often benefit from supportive and psychoeducational therapies.
   a. Psychoeducational approaches with families lead to decreased expression of anger and hostility within the family (so-called "expressed emotion"), which decreases relapse rates in schizophrenic patients.

III. Schizophreniform Disorder
   A. Manifests same acute symptoms as do persons with schizophrenia
   B. Total duration of all symptoms and functional impairment is only 1–6 months

C. Some patients go on to a subsequent psychotic relapse beyond the 1–6 month window, necessitating change in diagnosis to schizophrenia

D. This diagnostic category recognizes that some patients' psychoses are time-limited and reduces the potentially harmful "labeling" effects of a severe diagnosis such as schizophrenia

IV. Brief Psychotic Disorder

A. Catch-all rather than specific entity

B. Used to classify any brief (<1 month) episode of one or more psychotic symptoms

C. If associated with marked psychosocial stressors, corresponds to an older and still-used term, Brief Reactive Psychosis

D. Table 10.1 compares and contrasts Brief Psychotic Disorder with Schizophreniform Disorder and Schizophrenia

V. Schizoaffective Disorder

A. A heterogeneous "grab-bag" of presentations in the nebulous territory between schizophrenia and mood disorders

B. It may be that some persons with schizoaffective disorder really have schizophrenia (but with more prominent mood symptoms than most), whereas others may have a bad mood disorder (with more prominent psychotic symptoms than most) (Fig. 10.1)

 Older research diagnostic schemes used categories "schizoaffective, mainly schizophrenic" and "schizoaffective, mainly bipolar." These were unwieldy terms for everyday clinical use, yet they were instructive.

C. DSM IV-TR criteria for schizoaffective disorder stipulate that patient must have periods of psychosis *without* prominent mood symptoms *and* periods of full mood syndrome (manic or major depressive) concurrent with psychotic symptoms

 One can never diagnose schizoaffective disorder based on a single episode. There must be a history regarding at least two different types of episodes in order to diagnose.

TABLE 10.1	Comparison of Brief Psychotic and Schizophreniform Disorders With Schizophrenia VIII 7		
	Brief Psychotic Disorder	Schizophreniform Disorder	Schizophrenia
Duration of Symptoms	>1 day to <1 month	≥1 month to <6 months	≥6 months
Number of symptoms required of following list:	1 or more	2 or more*	2 or more*
Delusions	X	X	X
Hallucinations	X	X	X
Disorganized speech	X	X	X
Grossly disorganized or catatonic behavior	X	X	X
Negative symptoms	Not listed as criterion	X	X

*Only *one* symptom is required if delusions are bizarre, hallucinations consist of a voice keeping up a running commentary on the person's behavior or thoughts, or two or more voices converse with each other.

    D. Subtypes based on mood symptoms
       1. Depressive only
       2. Include periods of mania (bipolar type)
    E. Treatments
       1. Resemble treatments for schizophrenia and mood disorders
    F. Prognosis
       1. Quite variable
       2. Better when mood symptoms more prominent and poorer when psychotic symptoms more prominent

VI. Delusional Disorder
    A. Characteristic feature is *delusions* (stunning aptness of its name)
       1. Non-bizarre in nature (i.e., potentially plausible)
       2. Must be present for at least a month

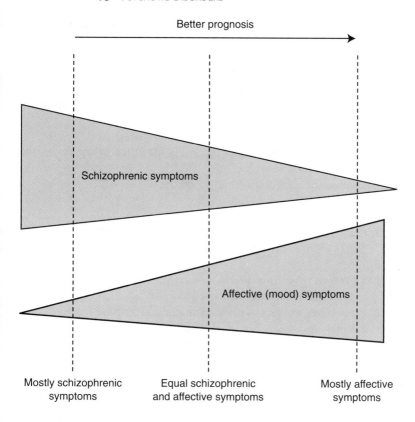

Better prognosis

Schizophrenic symptoms

Affective (mood) symptoms

| Mostly schizophrenic symptoms | Equal schizophrenic and affective symptoms | Mostly affective symptoms |

FIGURE 10.1 Spectrum of Schizoaffective Disorder.

   B. Thought process disorganization *not* found
   C. Hallucinations: either nonexistent or not prominent (although may
     be present if directly tied to delusional theme)
   D. Full criteria for schizophrenia not met
   E. Behavior and functioning not impaired except as related to
     delusional material
       1. No equivalents to negative symptoms of schizophrenia
   F. Several subtypes of delusional disorder described, based on
     predominant delusional theme
       1. Erotomanic (central theme: someone, usually famous or a supe-
       rior at work, is in love with the individual)

   2. Grandiose (central theme: conviction of having special powers, talents, or a special relationship with a prominent person or deity)

   3. Jealous (central theme: his or her spouse or lover is unfaithful)

   4. Persecutory (central theme: he or she is being spied on, conspired against, maligned, obstructed in some way)

   5. Somatic (central theme: abnormalities of body function or sensation)

   6. Mixed (no one delusional theme predominates)

   7. Unspecified (theme cannot be clearly identified or not among the subtypes listed above)

G. Uncommonly come to psychiatric attention

   1. Relative intactness of functioning

   2. Lack of insight into their illness

   3. Occasionally patients' actions lead to difficulties that cause others to force them to seek psychiatric care

H. Etiology

   1. Unknown (if known, would be secondary disorder, e.g., cocaine-induced delusional disorder)

   2. Neurobiological factors probably implicated but have received considerably less study than schizophrenia or major mood disorders

   3. Psychodynamic theories have focused on delusions' defensive usefulness as well as on symbolic meanings

I. Course

   1. Often chronic; some amount of waxing and waning may occur.

   2. A few patients have complete remission.

   3. Some patients may become increasingly preoccupied with the delusional system.

J. Treatment

   1. Maintaining a therapeutic alliance

> Maintaining a therapeutic alliance with patients with delusional disorder is no small task—by the nature of their disorder, they lack insight and tend to externalize rather than openly discuss their internal world.

   2. If compliance can be achieved: *antipsychotics* reduce the intensity of delusional preoccupation, even if not eliminate psychosis entirely

VII. Shared Psychotic Disorder
  A. Better known as *folie à deux* (French for "crazies of two")
  B. Patient with shared psychotic disorder comes to share delusions of another person (someone who has a psychotic disorder, usually schizophrenia)
  C. Usually patient has a close live-in relationship with this other person

 Shared Psychotic Disorder raises interesting questions about the relationships between environment and intrinsic diathesis (predisposition) toward psychosis.

  D. Rather uncommon
  E. Treatment
    1. Psychotropic medications
    2. Appropriate psychotherapeutic modalities

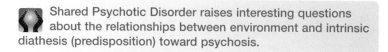

MENTOR TIPS DIGEST

- With psychotic *symptoms,* remember to think differential diagnosis.
- In differential diagnosis of psychotic symptoms, fundamentals remain such as careful medical history, physical examination including neurological exam, and basic laboratory tests.
- *Metabolic* issues tend to be focus of general health maintenance of patients on atypical antipsychotics, and *tardive dyskinesia* or *extrapyramidal symptoms* is the focus for patients on typical antipsychotics.
- Older research diagnostic scheme used categories "schizoaffective, mainly schizophrenic" and "schizoaffective, mainly bipolar." These were unwieldy terms for everyday clinical use, yet they were instructive.
- One can never diagnose schizoaffective disorder based on a single episode. There must be a history regarding at least two different types of episodes in order to diagnose.

- Maintaining a therapeutic alliance with patients with delusional disorder is no small task—by the nature of their disorder, they lack insight and tend to externalize rather than openly discuss their internal world.
- Shared Psychotic Disorder raises interesting questions about the relationships between environment and intrinsic diathesis (predisposition) toward psychosis.

Chapter Self-Test Questions

Circle the correct answer. After you have responded to the questions, check your answers in Appendix A.

1. Psychotic symptoms consist of hallucinations, delusions, and which of the following?
   a. Insomnia
   b. Negative symptoms
   c. Obsessions
   d. Thought-process disturbances

2. Which of the following disorders is associated with psychotic symptoms?
   a. Adjustment Disorder with Anxious Mood
   b. Adjustment Disorder with Depressed Mood
   c. Delirium
   d. Generalized Anxiety Disorder

3. One of the negative symptoms of schizophrenia is the lack of initiation of normal behaviors, such as grooming, dressing, seeking social interaction, and pursuing goal-directed tasks. This is called:
   a. Agnosis.
   b. Apraxia.
   c. Ataxia.
   d. Avolition.

4. Some patients with schizophrenia have a good prognosis, but others may be chronically symptomatic. Which of the following type of symptoms predicts the poorest outcome?

 a. Mood symptoms

 b. Negative symptoms

 c. Positive symptoms

 d. Ruminations

5. A 35-year-old man with schizophrenia was admitted to the surgical service after attempting to kill himself with a knife. He had heard voices telling him to kill himself, which he tried to suppress with drinking a half liter of vodka. He had been sober for 6 months prior to 1 month ago but had been drinking again regularly and increasingly over the last 4 weeks. Which of the following dispositions should follow his surgical hospitalization?

 a. Admission to a chemical dependency unit

 b. Admission to a MICA (dual diagnosis) inpatient unit

 c. Admission to a general psychiatric unit

 d. Outpatient follow-up with primary care provider, and Alcoholics Anonymous (AA) meetings.

See the testbank CD for more self-test questions.

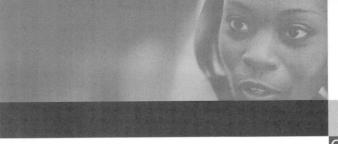

11

ANXIETY DISORDERS

**Michael R. Privitera, MD, MS, and
Jeffrey M. Lyness, MD**

I. Overview

    A. Anxiety is a hallmark symptom in this category.

    B. However, anxiety may be prominent in other "non-anxiety" disorders (e.g., delirium, dementia, mood disorders—especially depression and psychotic illnesses). **X7**

    C. Secondary anxiety disorders (i.e., due to general medical conditions or substance-induced) may demonstrate clinical features of generalized anxiety, panic attacks, obsessions, or compulsions. **X7**

    D. Anxiety from any cause is often associated with one or more somatic symptoms.

        1. May involve virtually every organ system and anatomic region (Table 11.1)

II. Panic Disorder

    A. Characterized by recurrent, unexpected, idiopathic panic attacks

    B. Panic attacks then followed by >1 month of worry about having another attack, about its consequences, or about change in behavior related to attacks (e.g., avoiding certain places for fear of having another attack) **X3**

    C. May occur with or without agoraphobia

    D. True panic attack

        1. Occurs over discrete period, for a few minutes to a few hours

        2. Anxiety present plus total of *four* (somatic) symptoms from Table 11.1 *or* psychological symptoms of:

            a. Derealization (feelings of unreality) or depersonalization (being detached from oneself)

            b. Fear of losing control or going crazy

            c. Fear of dying

TABLE 11.1	Physical Symptoms and Signs That May Be Associated With Anxiety X4
System	**Symptoms and Signs**
Cardiopulmonary	Chest pain Dyspnea Tachycardia Palpitations Elevated blood pressure
Autonomic	Diaphoresis Flushing Hot flashes or cold spells Dry mouth Pupillary mydriasis
Gastrointestinal	Nausea or vomiting Diarrhea Abdominal cramping or other pain Sense of dysphagia, choking, or "lump in the throat"
Neurological	Blurry vision Paresthesias (perioral, extremities) Tremor Dizziness or lightheadedness Muscle aches Gait unsteadiness
Genitourinary	Urinary urgency, frequency, or hesitancy

   3. Symptoms develop and increase rapidly; peak within 10 minutes
      a. Usually resolve in less than 1 hour
   E. Agoraphobia
      1. Anxiety about circumstances in which patient feels escape is difficult or help unavailable
      2. Typical circumstances are being alone outside one's home: alone in a crowd; on bridges, cars, buses, trains.

If fears of being outside one's home are limited to one specific situation, remember in differential diagnosis specific phobias as well as agoraphobia.

3. Patient avoids situations as above or endures them with considerable distress and fear of another attack or demands to be accompanied
4. May be part of a panic disorder (panic disorder with agoraphobia) or may exist alone (agoraphobia without history of panic disorder)

F. Panic disorder more prevalent in women—5% lifetime risk (compared with men: 2% lifetime risk) (X2)

G. Many patients presenting to general medical settings with specific somatic complaints have panic disorder

H. Course
   1. With treatment, most do well
   2. May have a chronic course, especially if maintenance treatments are discontinued

I. Treatment (see pathogenetic theories of anxiety disorders below for more on theoretical background to treatments) (X5)
   1. Cognitive/behavioral
      a. Psychotherapy focuses at first on *cognitive* misinterpretations of somatic symptoms (to break vicious cycle)
         i. Substituting more rational, hopeful interpretations → reduction in anxious affect
      b. After attacks reduced or eliminated, *behavioral* psychotherapeutic approaches used
         i. Help patient reengage with previously avoided situations (now they are safe and will not necessarily lead to panic attacks)
   2. Neurobiological (X1)
      a. Focuses on inappropriate or excessive activation of brain mediators of "fight or flight" response
      b. Treatment goal: dampen relevant neurobiological systems to reduce panic attacks
         i. Several antidepressants and fairly large doses of high-potency benzodiazepines, such as alprazolam or lorazepam

Although eventual dose of antidepressant drug used may be even higher than usual antidepressant doses, panic patients are highly sensitive to the initial anxiogenic effect of selective serotonin reuptake inhibitors (SSRIs) and other antidepressants. Hence, it is recommended to use ¼ to ½ of usual *initial* antidepressant dose (or less) when beginning treatment for such patients.

    c. Psychotherapy may also work by ultimately dampening hypersensitive or hyperactive neurobiological systems

  3. Most patients treated with combination of medications and blend of supportive, psychoeducational, and cognitive/behavioral psychotherapy

III. Phobias [X2]

A. Overview

  1. Are among the most common of mental disorders

  2. Vary in severity and consequence from relatively untroubling to entirely disabling

  3. Two major types: *specific* (or simple) phobias and *social* phobias

B. Specific (simple) phobias

  1. Fears of well-defined objects or situations (e.g., airplanes, heights, dogs)

  2. Attendant fear or avoidance phenomena must cause significant distress or affect patient's functioning or life routine

  3. Treatment

    a. Patient gradually exposed to series of situations that increasingly mimic his or her feared stimulus (*systematic desensitization,* based on learning theory as are all behavior therapies)

C. Social phobias

  1. Involve distressing or disabling fears of social or performance situations, in which patient is afraid that scrutiny or evaluation by others will lead to embarrassment or humiliation

  2. May be *circumscribed* (e.g., musician's "stage fright") or *generalized* to most social situations (in which case additional diagnosis of avoidant personality disorder should be considered)

  3. Treatment [X5]

    a. Cognitive/behavioral approaches (including desensitization and relaxation techniques) may have some value.

b. Pharmacotherapy (including monoamine oxidase inhibitors, SSRIs) has growing empirical support.
   i. Performance anxiety ("stage fright") may respond to these measures; beta-adrenergic blockers, when taken prior to performance, may help (probably by reducing sympathetically mediated anxiety symptoms such as tremor and palpitations).

IV. Obsessive-Compulsive Disorder X2
A. What obsessive-compulsive disorder (OCD) is *not*:
   1. "Obsessive," meaning rigidly preoccupied with details, to point of "not seeing forest for the trees"
   2. "To obsess" about something means preoccupied with worry about subject
   3. These definitions are accurate in and of themselves as applied to *obsessive-compulsive personality disorder* (discussed in Chapter 13)
B. OCD refers to much more specific symptoms
C. OCD may or may not occur in relation to obsessive-compulsive personality style or disorder
D. Persons with OCD suffer from either *obsessions* or *compulsions,* usually from both
   1. Obsessions and compulsions must cause significant distress, take up considerable time (more than 1 hour per day), or impair functioning
   2. *Obsessions:* recurrent mental activity, which may be thoughts, impulses, or images
      a. At some point, patients experience these as intrusive or inappropriate, so-called "ego-alien" (e.g., "I know these thoughts make no sense, but they keep popping up in my mind.").
      b. Many OCD patients may lose the ego-alien quality of their obsessions over time.
      c. To qualify as obsessions, thoughts, impulses, or images:
         i. Must not be simply worries about actual real-life problems.
         ii. Must not be solely a product of psychosis (e.g., delusions).
         iii. Must be the focus of efforts by the patient to "get rid" of them somehow, often by attempts at distraction or suppression.

    d. Typical obsessions are themes of contamination, doubts about past actions, a need for order or symmetry, and aggressive or sexual impulses, thoughts, or images.

    e. Often, patients describe a cycle of: annoying, ego-alien thoughts intrude on mind → attempts at suppression →→ mounting anxiety → abandon suppressive efforts → consequent relief of anxiety, but recurrence of unwanted obsession.

  3. *Compulsions:* in some sense are equivalent of obsessions in action; defined as repetitive behaviors (e.g., washing hands) or mental actions (e.g., counting)

    a. Patient feels driven to perform compulsive actions according to dictates of an obsession or some rigid, self-imposed rules.

    b. Patient's attempts to suppress compulsion lead to mounting anxiety.

    c. As occurs with ego-alien quality of obsession, patient recognizes that compulsions are unreasonable or excessive at some point during illness (although this may not be true for children).

E. Prevalence: OCD is more common than previously thought—about 1.5% (X2)

F. Course: tends to be chronic, and many patients with more severe forms of OCD are quite incapacitated by their symptoms

G. Treatment (X5)

  1. Psychodynamic perspectives

    a. Have had a longstanding field day with OCD

    b. Pay attention to symbolic meaning of individuals' specific obsessions and compulsions as unconscious mechanisms to manage what would otherwise be intolerable levels of anxiety

    c. Often lead to rich understanding of patient's mental life

    d. Psychodynamically-based psychotherapies have *not proved effective* in reducing obsessions or compulsions

  2. Pharmacotherapy

    a. Mainstays are SSRIs

    b. SSRI effectiveness has sparked interest in serotonergic-mediated disease mechanisms, but other neurotransmitters are probably also affected

    c. Other pharmacological agents alone or as adjuncts may be helpful in specific cases

      i. Clomipramine, monoamine oxidase inhibitors, lithium, antipsychotics, and anxiolytics

Clomipramine was the gold-standard drug for treatment of OCD; however, SSRIs' efficacy has been close enough that the more tolerable side-effect profiles have made them first-line treatment.

3. Behavioral therapies
   a. Reduce frequency of symptoms, particularly compulsive rituals
4. Cognitive-behavioral approaches using individual, group, or family modalities
   a. Are essential parts of comprehensive treatment of OCD patients
5. Psychosurgery—for severe and treatment-refractory OCD; treatments of last resort
   a. Ablative
      i. Stereotactically guided cingulotomy
   b. Neuromodulation
      i. Deep brain stimulation

V. Post-Traumatic Stress Disorder ✕2

A. Overview
1. Post-Traumatic Stress Disorder (PTSD) is a syndrome that arises in response to a psychologically traumatic event.
   a. Event: must be of greater magnitude than most encounter frequently
   b. DSM-IV defines "event" as one that threatens death or serious physical harm to self or others and that produces intense feelings of horror, fear, or helplessness
2. Not all persons exposed to such events—be they victims of rape, physical assault, warfare, or natural disaster—develop PTSD.
3. Possible outcomes from traumatic events are:
   a. PTSD.
   b. Depression.
   c. Other disorders (anxiety, mood, and psychotic disorders).
   d. Not enough symptoms to warrant diagnosis of a mental disorder at all.
4. Hence, there exists an interplay between external circumstances and a person's diathesis toward particular symptoms.
5. In PTSD, the proximate cause of disorder is a traumatic event: without the event, the person wouldn't have PTSD.

B. Diagnosis of PTSD, must have symptoms in *each of three realms*
  1. *"Positive or re-experiencing" symptoms:* recurrent and intrusive memories of event, dreams, event reenactments (which may include full-fledged flashback episodes), and worsening distress when exposed to stimuli that resemble event in some way
  2. *"Negative" symptoms: avoidance* (e.g., avoiding thoughts or discussions related to event; avoiding persons, activities, or places that are reminiscent of traumatic event; amnesia for part of event) and *numbing* phenomena (e.g., decreased interests, feeling detached from others, affective flattening, or sense of foreshortened future)
  3. Symptoms of *increased arousal:* insomnia, irritability, trouble concentrating, hypervigilance, or exaggerated startle response
C. If a limited but specific array of above present for 2 days to 1 month after traumatic event, DSM-IV assigns a diagnosis of Acute Stress Disorder; Table 11.2 compares and contrasts DSM-IV Acute Stress Disorder and PTSD
D. PTSD: if symptoms present for more than 1 month
  1. Subtypes are:
    a. *Acute* (up to 3 months)
    b. *Chronic* (longer than 3 months)
    c. *With delayed onset* (onset >6 months after event)
E. Only positive or re-experiencing symptoms are unique to PTSD
  1. Avoidance and hyperarousal symptoms may be seen in other anxiety disorders as well as mood disorders.
F. Course of PTSD may be complicated by full-fledged major depression or other disorders
  1. Comorbid diagnoses should be given and treated as appropriate.
G. Treatments (may profitably use several modalities)
  1. Empathetic relationship with individual psychotherapist
    a. Allows exploration of thoughts, images, and affects associated with traumatic event
    b. Such work is mainstay of treatment shortly after event happens (e.g., in acute stress disorder)—anxiolytics may also be helpful in short term
    c. These psychotherapeutic techniques helpful also for more chronic cases (establish treatment alliance within other modalities being used)
  2. Behavioral techniques may include relaxation training and exposure methods designed to reduce symptoms caused by cues associated with trauma

TABLE 11.2

Comparison of Acute Stress Disorder and PTSD [IX 6]

	Acute Stress Disorder	PTSD
Traumatic Event	Yes	Yes
Response: involves intense fear, helplessness, or horror	Yes	Yes
Dissociative signs or symptoms: (1) Numbing, detachment, emotional unresponsiveness (2) Decreased awareness of environment (3) Derealization (4) Depersonalization (5) Dissociative amnesia	≥3	—
Re-experiencing: recurrent images, thoughts, dreams, illusions, flashback episodes, sense of reliving experience, distress on reminders of trauma	≥1	≥1
Marked avoidance of stimuli that arouse recollections of trauma	Yes	Yes
Anxiety and ↑ arousal: difficulty sleeping, irritability, poor concentration, hypervigilance, exaggerated startle response	Yes or motor restlessness	≥2
Clinically significant distress or impairment	Yes	Yes
Duration of symptoms	2 days to 4 weeks	>1 month

Comparison of Acute Stress Disorder and PTSD **X6** (continued)		
	Acute Stress Disorder	**PTSD**
Not due to substance, medical condition, Brief Psychotic Disorder, or exacerbations of Axis I or II Disorder	Yes	—
Symptoms duration specifiers	—	*Acute:* 1–3 months *Chronic:* >3 months
Symptoms onset specifiers	—	None: if 2 days to 6 months after event *With delayed onset:* if >6 months after event

3. Medications should be used aggressively as indicated (and for comorbid syndromes as well, such as depression)
   a. Several classes of antidepressants may help with positive and hyperarousal symptoms of PTSD.
      i. Tricyclics
      ii. Monoamine oxidase inhibitors (MAOIs)
      iii. SSRIs
   b. Mood stabilizers have been tried but without clear guidelines.
   c. Alpha$_2$ agonists, such as clonidine and guanfacine, and alpha$_1$ antagonist prazosin have been used to reduce nightmares that persist.

Although it is not yet clear what the most effective means are to prevent progression of symptoms to acute stress disorder or PTSD after a traumatic event, early intervention with symptomatic control (e.g., improve sleep, reduce anxiety) and appropriate psychotherapy appear to be important.

4. Group psychotherapies for patients exposed to similar traumatic events can be a great help in acute and chronic variants of the disorder.

VI. Generalized Anxiety Disorder

A. Overview X2

1. Generalized Anxiety Disorder (GAD) is a relative "grab-bag" category of anxiety symptoms that do not quite fit any other anxiety or mood-disorder diagnosis.
2. Patient must have:
   a. >6 months of excessive anxiety or worry.
   b. At least three associated physical symptoms to an extent causing significant distress or dysfunction.
3. A large part of evaluation of such patients involves establishing that, in fact, anxiety is not better explained by a secondary anxiety disorder or other idiopathic syndrome (e.g., panic attacks, obsessions, depressive symptoms).
4. GAD may be most common of all anxiety disorders.
5. GAD often runs a chronic course.
6. GAD is commonly encountered in virtually all nonpsychiatric clinical settings.

B. Treatments X5

1. Psychotherapeutic
   a. Full continuum of psychodynamic psychotherapy
      i. From *expressive* (addressing more fundamental intrapsychic needs and conflicts) to *supportive* (emphasizing empathic alliance and stress management approaches)
      ii. Where along this continuum therapy should fall at any given time depends on variety of factors: patient's personality style; his or her strengths and vulnerabilities (including personality pathology); his or her capacity to form an interpersonal alliance with therapist; degree of symptomatology at time; nature of therapeutic setting (e.g., short- vs. long-term frequency of visits)
   b. Cognitive and behavioral techniques
      i. May be useful, paralleling their use in panic disorder
2. Pharmacotherapy
   a. Benzodiazepines: usually for short-term use but may be long-term if other options not helpful

    b. Buspirone: has been useful mainstay in chronic setting without the addictive potential of benzodiazepines

    c. Some serotonin-norepinephrine reuptake inhibitors (SNRI) and SSRI antidepressants: have shown superior efficacy to buspirone

    d. Tricyclics: efficacy in GAD independent of effect on panic attacks and depressive symptoms not clear

VII. Pathogenetic Theories of Anxiety Disorders ⓧ🄵

  A. Usual biopsychosocial gamut

  B. Psychodynamics

    1. Early traditions: anxiety is hallmark of unresolved unconscious conflict

    2. More recent schools (e.g., built around object-relations theory): proneness to unpleasant affects and fears results from lack of internal sense of whole self

      a. Leads to inability to soothe oneself without direct support from other people (see Chapter 13)

    3. OCD notoriously *not* responsive to psychodynamic psychotherapy

    4. PTSD symptoms may be understood as:

      a. Attempt to master the "unmasterable."

      b. Learned responses to cues associated with original trauma.

  C. Cognitive/behavioral psychology

    1. Many anxiety reactions understood as catastrophic misinterpretations of normal bodily sensation, which initiates a downward cascade

      a. Anxiety → more somatic symptoms → more anxiety

    2. Anticipatory anxiety and avoidance

      a. Understood as learned behaviors in response to anxiety

  D. Social

    1. Effects of anxiety disorders on family may be far-reaching.

    2. Early life separations are risk factor for later anxiety.

    3. Family attempts to help may perpetuate symptoms (learning theory) (e.g., use of family companions for panic or altering family life to allow OCD patient to perform compulsions).

  E. Neurobiology

    1. Panic Disorder and PTSD

      a. Central nucleus of *amygdala* coordinates neurobiological response

    i. *Inputs:* excitatory glutamatergic, from cortical sensory areas and thalamus

    ii. *Outputs* to:

        (1) Norepinephrine neurons of locus coeruleus

        (2) Dopamine neurons of ventral tegmental area

        (3) Serotonin neurons of raphe nuclei

    iii. Central nucleus can orchestrate multiple aspects of anxiety disorders

        (1) Cognitive misappraisal/fear (cortex)

        (2) Escape or freezing behavior (periaqueductal gray)

        (3) Other motor activation (striatum)

        (4) Hyperventilation (parabrachial nucleus)

        (5) Sympathetic activation (lateral hypothalamus)

        (6) Gastrointestinal (GI) distress (dorsal motor nucleus of vagus)

        (7) Exaggerated startle response (nucleus caudalis pontis)

b. Neuroendocrine

    i. Increased corticotropin-releasing factor (CRF) "stress response" in:

        (1) hypothalamo-portal system

        (2) projections from central nucleus of amygdala

c. Gamma-aminobutyric acid (GABA)

    i. Most "anxiolytics" work by enhancing GABA (inhibitory) function

        (1) GABA distributed widely; acts on many of above systems

        (2) GABA inhibits corticotropin-releasing factor (CRF) from paraventricular nucleus in hypothalamus

d. Altered central and peripheral noradrenergic function may mediate hyperarousal of PTSD

2. OCD

a. Prominent frontal and striatal mechanisms

b. Powerful role for serotonin systems and serotonergic drugs in therapy

c. Possibly akin to animal grooming behaviors (inappropriate institution of preprogrammed neural scripts?)

d. Genetic: probably related to tic syndromes, such as Tourette's disorder

MENTOR TIPS DIGEST

- If fears of being outside one's home are limited to one specific situation, remember in differential diagnosis specific phobias as well as agoraphobia.
- Although the eventual dose of antidepressant drug used may be even higher than usual antidepressant doses, panic patients are highly sensitive to the initial anxiogenic effect of SSRIs. Hence, it is recommended to use ¼ to ½ of usual *initial* antidepressant dose (or less) when beginning treatment for such patients.
- Clomipramine was the gold-standard drug for treatment of OCD; however, SSRIs' efficacy has been close enough that the more tolerable side-effect profiles have made them first-line treatment.
- Although it is not yet clear what the most effective means are to prevent progression of symptoms to acute stress disorder or PTSD after a traumatic event, early intervention with symptomatic control (e.g., improve sleep, reduce anxiety) and appropriate psychotherapy appear to be important.

Chapter Self-Test Questions

Circle the correct answer. After you have responded to the questions, check your answers in Appendix A.

1. Which nucleus has been implicated in coordinating the neurobiological response in panic disorder and PTSD?

   a. Accumbens

   b. Amygdala

   c. Caudalis pontis

   d. Gracilis

2. Which of the following cardiopulmonary symptoms is most closely associated with anxiety?

   a. Chest pain

   b. Dyspnea on exertion

c. Nocturia

d. Orthopnea

3. Which of the following autonomic symptoms is most closely associated with anxiety?

a. Bradycardia

b. Diastolic hypertension

c. Flushing

d. Orthostatic hypotension

4. A 38-year-old bank executive just lost his job due to downsizing and presents to the emergency unit with chest pain, tachycardia, dyspnea, paresthesias in his arms and hands, fear of losing his mind, and feelings of unreality. Physical examination, electrocardiogram, cardiac enzymes, and troponins are all negative. His most likely diagnosis is which of the following?

a. Adjustment Disorder with Anxious Mood

b. Anxiety Disorder NOS

c. Histrionic Personality Disorder

d. Myocardial infarction

5. A 55-year-old woman with a history of panic attacks had an attack spontaneously when at the park in her neighborhood. Since that time, she has been unwilling to leave her apartment alone and insists on having a family member with her. Which of the following is the most likely diagnosis?

a. Adjustment Disorder with Anxious Mood

b. Avoidant personality disorder

c. Histrionic personality disorder

d. Panic disorder with agoraphobia

See the testbank CD for more self-test questions!

12
CHAPTER

SUBSTANCE USE DISORDERS

Michael R. Privitera, MD, MS, and Jeffrey M. Lyness, MD

I. Overview

A. History, sociology, economics, pharmacology, and other aspects of substance use disorders have made many a fine book and are well beyond this book's scope.

B. In United States, substance use disorders are the most prevalent of all mental disorders. **VII 3**

    1. Enormous consequences for U.S. population's mental and physical health **VII 9**

    2. Tremendous consequences affecting society as a whole **VII 9**

C. No physician will escape encountering myriad effects of substance use disorders on patients, their families, and communities.

II. Concepts and Definitions

A. DSM-IV-TR classification of "substance-related disorders" can seem confusing

B. Following concepts may make principles of classification more straightforward:

    1. Each *substance class* is listed separately (Box 12.1).

    2. Under substance class you will find several possible types of disorders. **VII 2** (Table 12.1; Figs. 12.1 and 12.2)

        a. *Intoxications:* substance-specific, reversible, maladaptive behavioral states caused by having drug "on board"

        b. *Withdrawal states:* substance-specific maladaptive conditions caused by reduction or cessation of intake of substance

        c. *Cognitive disorders:* due to intoxication or withdrawal involving a specific substance (e.g., alcohol withdrawal delirium, dementia)

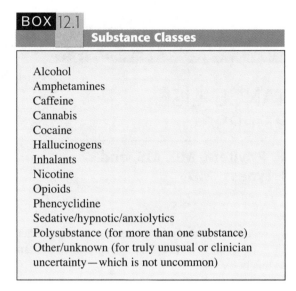

BOX 12.1

Substance Classes

Alcohol
Amphetamines
Caffeine
Cannabis
Cocaine
Hallucinogens
Inhalants
Nicotine
Opioids
Phencyclidine
Sedative/hypnotic/anxiolytics
Polysubstance (for more than one substance)
Other/unknown (for truly unusual or clinician uncertainty—which is not uncommon)

    d. Specific mental syndromes *caused by substance,* called *substance-induced disorders,* resembling secondary syndromes (e.g., substance-induced psychotic, mood, anxiety, or sleep disorders; and sexual dysfunctions)

  3. Some disorders relate to pattern of misuse of substance.

    a. It is possible to have a substance-induced mental disorder or state of intoxication *without* having a history of abuse.

    b. Most patients with intoxication or other substance-induced disorder have recurrent substance use; these conditions with problematic use are termed *substance-use disorders.*

III. Substance Dependence Versus Abuse VII 2

  A. DSM-IV defines two kinds of substance use syndromes

    1. Substance Dependence

      a. At least three of following physiological and behavioral phenomena must occur in a 12-month period.

        i. Tolerance (more drug needed to obtain same effect)

        ii. Withdrawal (either characteristic withdrawal syndrome for the substance or same or closely related substance is taken to prevent or treat withdrawal symptoms)

TABLE 12.1
Examples From Some Substance Classes

Class	Examples
Sedative-Hypnotics	Barbiturates Meprobamate Chloral hydrate Alcohol Benzodiazepines Nonbenzodiazepines (e.g., zolpidem)
Stimulants	Amphetamine Cocaine Methylphenidate
Opioids	Heroin Methadone Morphine Pentazocine
Dissociatives	Ketamine Phencyclidine (PCP)
Psychedelics	Lysergic acid diethylamide (LSD) Mescaline Psilocybin
Anticholinergics	Benztropine Diphenhydramine Hydroxyzine

iii. Substance taken in larger amounts or longer time than was planned

iv. Attempts to cut down or somehow modify substance use pattern

v. Much time spent in getting, using, or recovering from substance

vi. Reduction of time spent in other, nonsubstance-related activities

vii. Continues substance use despite patient's knowledge of adverse consequences (which may range from depression to marital conflict to physical sequelae such as alcohol-associated gastritis)

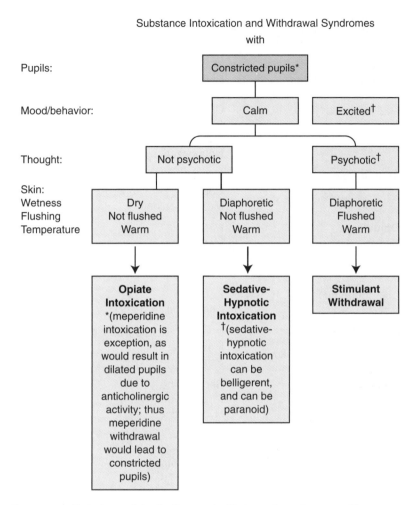

FIGURE 12.1 Substance intoxication and withdrawal syndromes with constricted pupils. VII 10

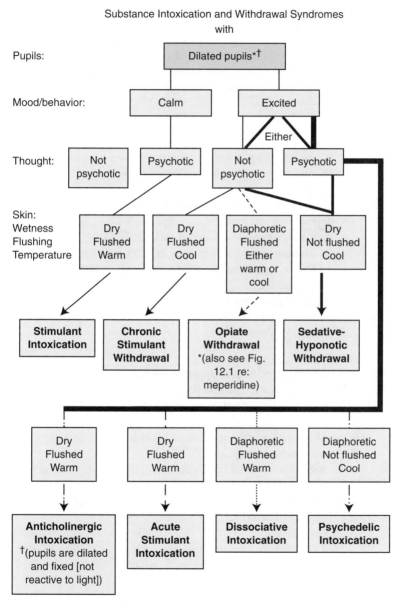

FIGURE 12.2 Substance intoxication and withdrawal syndromes with dilated pupils.

Physiological dependence alone is not sufficient to be diagnosed with the mental disorder "substance dependence." Any patient can develop drug tolerance and withdraw if the drug (like an opioid) is stopped suddenly. If the drug is taken as prescribed, and it does not adversely affect the patient's life, then the patient does not suffer from a substance use disorder.

2. Substance Abuse:
   a. Is a lesser, but still potentially devastating, disorder involving an adverse psychological or social consequence related to substance use.
   b. Is lesser because the diagnosis is *not* given if criteria for dependence are met.
   c. Adverse consequences might include: (VII 4)
      i. Impairment in performance at work or home.
      ii. Use in hazardous situations (e.g., driving while intoxicated).
      iii. Legal problems related to substance use.
      iv. Continued use despite adverse effects on interpersonal relationships.

IV. Etiology (VII 8)
   A. Although many principles apply broadly across all drugs, many factors are unique to specific drugs.
   B. A breadth of factors need to be considered
      1. Genetics
         a. Plays a clear role in some addictions, particularly alcoholism
      2. Neuropharmacology
         a. Mediates some of reinforcing qualities of intoxication (e.g., pleasurable high of cocaine)
         b. Mediates unpleasant qualities of withdrawal states (reinforcing continued drug use)
      3. Neurobiology
         a. Dopamine reward pathway reinforces "high" of most drugs
         b. Nucleus accumbens ("pleasure center")
      4. Other neurobiological factors
         a. Individual susceptibility to dependence on particular drugs (e.g., persons with attention deficit disorder and their paradoxical relaxation with cocaine or other stimulants)

5. Psychological perspectives
    a. Psychological usefulness (and therefore positive reinforcement) of drug effects ("self-medication hypothesis")
        i. Modulate unpleasant affects
        ii. Regulate impulse control
        iii. Other psychological functions (that healthier persons would manage without drug use)
6. Psychosocial factors
    a. Cultural expectations affect:
        i. Choice of drugs.
        ii. Prevalence rates.
        iii. Patterns of use (e.g., binge drinking versus chronic moderate drinking).
    b. "Culture" (in this context) includes:
        i. Families.
        ii. Ethnic groups.
        iii. Religious affiliations.
        iv. Subcultural identifications.
        v. Nationalities.
    c. Prevalence affected by factors such as drug availability, cost, legal risks, and other risks

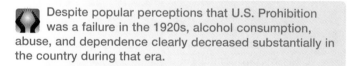
Despite popular perceptions that U.S. Prohibition was a failure in the 1920s, alcohol consumption, abuse, and dependence clearly decreased substantially in the country during that era.

V. Treatment ⬚VII 6⬚

A. Wide range of alternatives to use (given variety of pathogenetic backgrounds)
B. Drugs may be used singly, but more often in combination
C. Many treatments are socially-based approaches that are separate from treatments offered by medical professionals (although hopefully there is cooperation between the two approaches)
    1. Goals: to maintain abstinence and foster a sense of interpersonal (and often spiritual) connectedness in a drug-free context
    2. Alcoholics Anonymous (AA): most prominent of socially-based approaches
    3. Other self-help groups based on 12-step or similar philosophies

D. Many other community, church, or other social organizations may be of use, providing support and social connectedness

E. Medically based addiction programs offer range of services
1. Inpatient detoxification
2. Rehabilitation
3. Day treatment programs
4. Less intensive varieties of outpatient contacts

F. Group, family, and individual psychotherapies tend to focus on:
1. Breaking down (often prominent) denial.
2. Breaking down "enabling" behavior by family and friends.
3. Identifying social or intrapsychic cues that signal or provoke impending relapse to drug use.
4. Building comprehensive strategies to minimize such provocations.
5. Managing patient's dysphoric or otherwise mental states without using drugs.

G. Pharmacotherapy
1. May play a role in many specific drug dependencies, even beyond role in detoxification (examples)
   a. Reduction of reward
      i. Naltrexone for alcoholism
      ii. Varenicline (Chantix) for cigarette smoking
   b. Reduction of craving
      i. Acamprosate (Campral): stimulates GABA-ergic neurotransmission and antagonizes glutamate
      ii. Transdermal/gum/lozenge nicotine for cigarette smoking
      iii. Methadone for opioids
   c. Negative reinforcer
      i. Disulfiram (Antabuse) for alcohol use

H. Nearly all treatment programs with documented efficacy aim for total abstinence as goal

> Occasionally, addicted individuals may be able to achieve a state of "controlled drinking" (i.e., use at non-abuse, nondependent levels), *but most cannot*. Aiming for anything less than full abstinence usually results in colluding with their denial about the severity of their disorder.

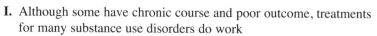

I. Although some have chronic course and poor outcome, treatments for many substance use disorders do work

    1. Large numbers of people benefit from these interventions.

J. Aggressive treatment of comorbid psychopathology (e.g., mood or anxiety disorders) likely to improve outcome for patients with substance dependence

 MENTOR TIPS DIGEST

- *Physiological dependence* alone is not sufficient to be diagnosed with the mental disorder "substance dependence". Any patient can develop drug tolerance and withdraw if the drug (like an opioid) is stopped suddenly. If the drug is taken as prescribed, and it does not adversely affect the person's life, then the patient does not suffer from a substance use disorder.
- Despite popular perceptions that U.S. Prohibition was a failure in the 1920s, alcohol consumption, abuse, and dependence clearly decreased substantially in the country during that era.
- Occasionally, addicted individuals may be able to achieve a state of "controlled drinking" (i.e., use at non-abuse, nondependent levels), *but most cannot.* Aiming for anything less than full abstinence usually results in colluding with their denial about the severity of their disorder.

Resources

Giannini AJ: An Approach to Drug Abuse, Intoxication and Withdrawal. American Family Physician 61:2763–2774, 2000.

Chapter Self-Test Questions

Circle the correct answer. After you have responded to the questions, check your answers in Appendix A.

1. In the United States which of the following are the most prevalent of all mental disorders?

a. Anxiety Disorders

b. Mood Disorders

c. Schizophrenic Disorders

d. Substance Use Disorders

2. A substance-specific, reversible, maladaptive behavioral state caused by having a drug on board is called:

a. Delirium.

b. Encephalopathy.

c. Intoxication.

d. Withdrawal.

3. A 38-year-old man presented to the emergency department with a 3-day history of insomnia, paranoia, and auditory hallucinations. He is fully oriented, and his memory and attention are intact. His family history is negative for psychiatric conditions; he is on no prescribed medications; and his wife confirms that he has never gone through symptoms like this. He has been socializing with new acquaintances from work, which she felt were not in his best interests. His urine toxicology screen came back positive for amphetamines. His most likely diagnosis is:

a. Delirium due to amphetamines.

b. Schizophrenia.

c. Schizophreniform disorder.

d. Substance-induced psychotic disorder.

4. A 42-year-old female with a seizure disorder has been treated with phenobarbital. She takes her medicine as prescribed, and the medication does not impair her in her usual life functioning. She went away for the weekend with her husband but forgot her medications. On Sunday morning, she began to get symptoms and signs of being shaky, tachycardic, dilated pupils and highly anxious until she resumed her medication when she arrived home Sunday evening. Her most likely diagnosis is:

a. Adjustment disorder with anxious mood.

b. Anxiety disorder NOS.

c. Physiological dependence on phenobarbital.

d. Sedative dependence disorder.

5. A drug used in the treatment of alcohol dependence that works by reducing craving is:

    a. Acamprosate.

    b. Disulfiram.

    c. Naltrexone.

    d. Varenicline.

See the testbank CD for more self-test questions.

13

PERSONALITY TRAITS AND DISORDERS

Michael R. Privitera, MD, MS, and Jeffrey M. Lyness, MD

I. Overview

A. "Personality" is a complex, elusive, and allusive term.

B. In the interest of educational clarity, personality in a broad sense refers to a person's enduring patterns of thinking, feeling, acting, and reacting.

1. "Enduring" implies fundamentally stable throughout life (empirical research has shown that various measures of personality mostly do remain stable across the lifespan).

2. Nevertheless, important changes in personality are possible.

   a. Facilitated by desired or undesired life events, psychotherapy, or other experiences

3. By current schemes of psychopathology, personality is considered the backdrop to development of Axis I psychiatric disorders covered thus far.

   a. Sometimes an *active backdrop*
      i. Certain personality styles or structures may put an individual at higher risk for specific psychopathology.

   b. Sometimes a *passive backdrop*
      i. Certain personality styles or structures color the patient's perspectives and reactions to illness and affect relationships with caregivers and providers.

C. The *Diagnostic and Statistical Manual of Mental Disorders* (DSM-IV-TR) continues the distinction between personality and other psychopathology. **XVI 1**

1. In multiaxial diagnostic scheme placed on Axis II, where other psychiatric diagnoses except mental retardation is placed on Axis I

The distinction between Axis II and I can be useful but sometimes arbitrary and difficult or impossible to make. For example, lifelong chronic depressive or anxiety symptoms become inseparably intertwined with personality. Therefore, it is important to accept this possible coexistence and treat symptomatic manifestations as best as possible.

D. Acute mental states may alter what appears to be personality. [XVI 7]
1. A person with severe major depression may be needy, clingy, and dependent on others for support and reassurance but does not have dependent personality style when not depressed.
2. Many psychologically healthy people regress to using more rigid and dysfunctional defense mechanisms under acute stress, such as severe acute medical illness.

 Beware of diagnosing or labeling patients with personality disorder *solely* on how they appear to you *now*. Dysfunctional patterns need to be enduring rather than artifacts of patients' current state.

E. Most prominent and clinically useful perspectives on understanding personality disorders are psychodynamic and developmentally based. [XVI 3]
1. Personality understood to develop in childhood from interplay between constitutional factors (genetic and prenatal influences) and life experiences
   a. Life experiences include obvious stressors or traumatic events as well as nuances of quality of relationships with others (parents and other primary caregivers)
   b. Interplay goes *both ways*—inborn temperament can shape responses elicited from others (e.g., harder to be consistently calm and loving parent with a constitutionally irritable and inconsolable baby)
F. A patient's current personality structure can be understood by using metapsychological frameworks (e.g., psychodynamics) regarding the patient's:
1. Common ways of perceiving others and the world
2. Repertoire of problem-solving strategies
3. Predominant defense mechanisms
4. Patterns of regulating and expressing affects and impulses

G. Labels may be useful in describing these personality characteristics (traits).

1. Derived from psychodynamic descriptions
   a. Schizoid
   b. Narcissistic
   c. Obsessive
2. Other schemes of how many or how few traits an individual has—more helpful in research than clinical work
3. Linking fundamental traits with neurobiological function (e.g., novelty seeking with dopaminergic activity)—translation into clinical practice still remains elusive

II. DSM-IV-TR Definitions XVI 1

A. Everyone has personality *traits,* but some people have a constellation of traits that cause particular difficulty.

B. Personality Disorders are defined by DSM-IV-TR as existing when personality:

1. Deviates markedly from cultural expectations.
2. Is inflexible and pervasive across a broad range of situations.
3. Causes subjective distress or impairment in interpersonal relationships or other role functioning (e.g., work, school).

C. DSM-IV-TR describes a number of subtypes of personality disorders based on relatively external, observable, reproducible criteria sets.

1. Advantages of this approach
   a. High degree of inter-rater reliability in diagnosis
   b. Many resulting diagnoses appear to be clinically meaningful; have relatively specific epidemiology, course, and treatment responses
2. Disadvantages of this approach
   a. Clinical richness lacking as compared with, e.g., psychodynamic formulations
   b. Some entities may not be as meaningful as others
   c. Many persons with clearly disordered personalities cannot be usefully categorized by single DSM-IV-TR diagnosis

Given the disadvantages of DSM-IV-TR's categories of personality disorders, it is not surprising that clinicians need to use a variety of perspectives beyond DSM-ese to understand and work with patients with personality difficulties.

D. Still, it is worth becoming familiar with basic outlines of DSM-IV-TR personality disorders. They are grouped as three clusters. **XVI 2**
  1. Not Otherwise Specified (NOS) is used for individuals who meet criteria for personality disorder, but not a specific DSM type.
  2. Other types of personality disorders have been described, with criteria suggested, such as are found in the DSM-IV-TR appendix.
    a. Depressive Personality Disorder
    b. Passive-Aggressive Personality Disorder
  3. Brief descriptions of DSM-IV-TR disorders follow.
E. Cluster A (Odd or Eccentric)
  1. Schizoid Personality Disorder
    a. Appear eccentric because of affective detachment and emotional coldness
    b. Socially isolated by choice because they do not desire or seek closeness with others
    c. May function well in occupational settings (typically in jobs that require little interpersonal contact or skills) but otherwise choose to lead largely solitary lives
    d. Because of above characteristics, rarely have subjective distress or chaotic interpersonal function that leads to psychiatric contact
    e. Manifestations resemble prodromal or negative symptoms of schizophrenia

> A person with schizoid personality may later receive a diagnosis of schizophrenia if individual goes on to develop frank psychotic symptoms, but many persons have stable schizoid personalities throughout their lives without developing psychotic illness.

  2. Schizotypal Personality Disorder
    a. Also appear eccentric but in a more flamboyant way
    b. Have oddities of thinking and speech, unusual ideas or beliefs, and either constricted or inappropriate affect
    c. Tend to be socially isolated, sometimes by preference, sometimes simply because their eccentricities drive others away, or become fearful in social settings
    d. By definition, unusual thought processes and content to not reach frankly psychotic proportions

Persons with schizotypal personality disorder are probably at higher risk of becoming psychotic under stress; at which point an additional Axis I diagnosis would be given to appropriately describe the psychotic syndrome. **XVI 8**

3. Paranoid Personality Disorder
   a. Have paranoid thoughts; i.e., are distrustful and suspicious of others
   b. Paranoia is *not* of delusional intensity

Persons with paranoid personality disorder may be more likely than others to become flagrantly psychotic at times of stress; an additional diagnosis of appropriate psychotic disorder would be made. **XVI 8**

F. Cluster B (Dramatic, Emotional, or Erratic)
   1. Borderline Personality Disorder
      a. Fundamental underlying characteristics generated from psychodynamic perspectives that led to recognition and definition of borderline personality disorder
         i. Lack of sense of self (not simply low self-esteem—genuine absence of whole, integrated self-image)
         ii. Use of primitive, maladaptive defense mechanisms such as splitting, projection, and projective identification
      b. Term "borderline" comes from object-relations theory; refers to intermediate position of such personality structure between healthier "neurotic" and more impaired "psychotic" personality organizations.
      c. More directly observable criteria of DSM-IV-TR for borderline personality disorder
         i. Recurrent chaotic interpersonal relationships
         ii. Extreme sensitivity to real or perceived abandonment
         iii. Evidence of identity disturbance
         iv. Chronic feelings of emptiness
         v. Affective instability (lifelong shifts between extremes of mood states) or frequent expressions of anger
         vi. Self-destructive impulsivity

vii. Repeated or chronic suicidal ideation or directly self-injurious actions

viii. Transient psychotic symptoms (including paranoid delusions or hallucinations) during periods of stress

  d. Spectrum of functionality

  i. Healthier end: persons with borderline personality may maintain jobs and long-term relationships with others, albeit with considerable subjective distress and interpersonal turmoil under the functional surface

  ii. More severe forms: often high utilizers of psychiatric (and medical) services, often forming difficult, chaotic relationships with caregivers

> In working with patients with borderline personality disorder, considerable affect can often be evoked in caregivers. The caregiver must monitor this affect carefully to provide appropriate, professional, effective treatments. **XVI 11**

2. Narcissistic Personality Disorder

  a. Most prominent features

  i. Evidence of grandiosity of thoughts or behavior

  ii. Need for recognition for self-perceived specialness

  iii. Lack of empathy for others

  b. Persons with this disorder often meet criteria for other personality disorders

  i. Psychodynamic perspective: hollow core underneath grandiose bluster of pathological narcissism

  ii. Many persons with this disorder have borderline personality-type organization

  (1) Concomitant lack of sense of self

  (2) Propensity for primitive, maladaptive defenses

  c. Unlike "pure" borderline personalities, narcissistic persons cover up their borderline core with shell of grandiosity

  d. "Cover" has advantages

  i. Narcissistic personalities much less prone to affective instability, poor impulse control, or suicidal tendencies than are "pure" borderline personalities

  e. BUT—grandiose shell thin and hollow

    i. Requires constant reinforcement to keep intact

    ii. Interpersonal relationships viewed solely in terms of how much they help maintain grandiose image by admiration, recognition of specialness

3. Antisocial Personality Disorder

    a. Cardinal feature: pervasive disregard for and violation of rights of others

    b. More common in men

    c. Prevalent in prison populations

    d. Often comorbid with substance-use disorders

    e. Manifestations

        i. Chronic lying or other deceitfulness

        ii. Law breaking

        iii. Irresponsibility

        iv. Aggressiveness

        v. Novelty-seeking actions (with disregard for safety of self or others)

        vi. Lack of remorse

        vii. Externalizing blame

    f. Must show evidence of conduct disorder before age 15 years (manifestations being essentially childhood equivalents of adult antisocial behaviors)

    g. Referred to as *sociopaths* or *psychopaths* in lay media

    h. Can appear charismatically charming or ingratiating if doing so serves their immediate needs

    i. Often appear to be wholly without anxiety or worries of any sort

    j. Beneath surface of smoothness and confidence is sense of *emptiness*; not easily apparent as relationships with others tend to be brief and superficial

    k. Treatment

        i. Unlikely to benefit from treatment by traditional psychiatric settings and methods (by definition, relationships with others are usually built around exploitation to gratify immediate needs)

4. Histrionic Personality Disorder

    a. Main characteristics: excessive emotionality (theatrical) and attention seeking

    b. Despite striking displays of affect, often superficial quality to emotional life and relationships

   c. Manifestations
     i. Suggestible
     ii. Impulsive in beliefs and actions
     iii. Flirtatious or otherwise sexually provocative styles often used to help draw attention to self
     iv. Spectrum of severity
       (1) Healthier end: retain capacity for relatively unambivalent intimacy
         (A) Allows them to make more successful use of psychodynamic psychotherapy
       (2) More severe end: histrionic style may be underlined by fundamental troubles with sense of self (i.e., borderline personality organization)
         (A) Greater difficulties in interpersonal relationships, including psychotherapies

G. Cluster C (Anxious or Fearful)
   1. Avoidant Personality Disorder
     a. Core feature: pattern of social inhibition, related to feelings of inadequacy; fears of being criticized, shamed, or rejected
     b. Considerable overlap with generalized social phobia; often both diagnoses apply—may be same or similar conditions

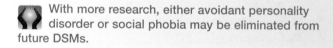

With more research, either avoidant personality disorder or social phobia may be eliminated from future DSMs.

     c. Social phobia defined more narrowly (i.e., anxiety while actually facing social situations)
     d. Avoidant personality disorder defined in terms of broader preoccupations with self-image as related to others
   2. Dependent Personality Disorder
     a. Core features: excessive need to be taken care of, leading to submissive, clinging behavior and fear of being left alone
     b. Dependent behaviors common in other personality disorders and other disorders, such as major depression
       i. Dependency features pervasive and enduring (e.g., present not only when patient is depressed XVI 6)
       ii. More specific neediness of other personality disorders (e.g., narcissists requiring admiration) lacking

3. Obsessive-Compulsive Personality Disorder
   a. Demonstrate preoccupation with details, orderliness, and perfectionism as means to maintaining control over mental activity and interpersonal events

> Here the term "obsessiveness" retains its familiar meaning from lay usage, different from the *obsessions* of obsessive-compulsive disorder. Keep in mind that some degree of obsessiveness is useful to completing tasks and achieving goals.

   b. Obsessiveness at expense of flexibility, openness, and efficiency.
      i. Major point of activities may be lost
      ii. Tasks may not be completed
      iii. Relationships beyond those needed for work and productivity often impaired
4. Passive-Aggressive Personality Disorder
   a. Not an official DSM-IV-TR diagnosis
      i. Listed in DSM-IV-TR appendix as criteria set for further study.
   b. Concept of passive-aggressive style worth mentioning because it is common and troubling dynamic seen in persons with other personality disorders (and some without)
   c. Characterized by pervasive pattern of negativistic attitudes and passive resistance to demands for adequate performance
   d. Typically, combination of passively failing to complete tasks (e.g., by "forgetting" or indefinite procrastination) along with tendency to blame others and deny responsibility for lack of accomplishments

> Persons with passive-aggressive personality disorder control their lives and environment through inaction.

H. Figure 13.1 is a flowchart that illustrates diagnostic reasoning regarding personality disorders.

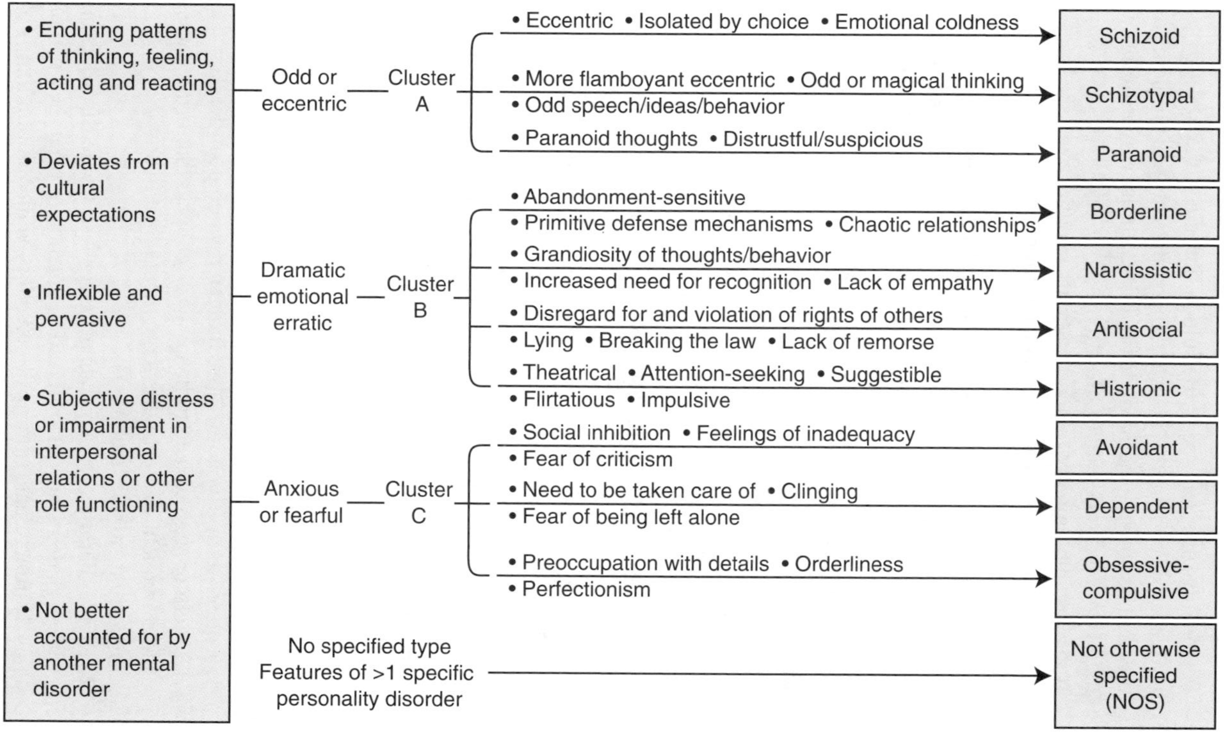

FIGURE 13.1 Personality disorder diagnostic flowchart. XVI 1

Flowchart content:

Left box:
- Enduring patterns of thinking, feeling, acting and reacting
- Deviates from cultural expectations
- Inflexible and pervasive
- Subjective distress or impairment in interpersonal relations or other role functioning
- Not better accounted for by another mental disorder

Cluster A — Odd or eccentric
- Eccentric • Isolated by choice • Emotional coldness → Schizoid
- More flamboyant eccentric • Odd or magical thinking • Odd speech/ideas/behavior → Schizotypal
- Paranoid thoughts • Distrustful/suspicious → Paranoid

Cluster B — Dramatic emotional erratic
- Abandonment-sensitive • Primitive defense mechanisms • Chaotic relationships → Borderline
- Grandiosity of thoughts/behavior • Increased need for recognition • Lack of empathy → Narcissistic
- Disregard for and violation of rights of others • Lying • Breaking the law • Lack of remorse → Antisocial
- Theatrical • Attention-seeking • Suggestible • Flirtatious • Impulsive → Histrionic

Cluster C — Anxious or fearful
- Social inhibition • Feelings of inadequacy • Fear of criticism → Avoidant
- Need to be taken care of • Clinging • Fear of being left alone → Dependent
- Preoccupation with details • Orderliness • Perfectionism → Obsessive-compulsive

No specified type
Features of >1 specific personality disorder → Not otherwise specified (NOS)

185

III. Treatment XVI 9

A. Personality disorders are by definition chronic.

B. By nature of personality disorder, many patients see problems as the faults of others and have difficulty accepting responsibility for their own recurrent pattern of action.

C. If less psychologically minded, patients may not even see a recurrent pattern, let alone understand their role in perpetuating it.

> In many quarters, treatment of personality disorders has a rather hopeless reputation. Empirical research has shown that personality usually remains remarkably stable throughout adulthood. Yet, being realistic about prognosis does not mean feeling hopeless.

D. Most persons in psychiatric settings with personality disorders are suffering from a comorbid Axis I disorder.
   1. Common comorbidities
      a. Mood disorders
      b. Anxiety disorders
      c. Substance use disorders
      d. Adjustment disorders
   2. Aggressive treatment of comorbid Axis I disorder essential and helpful in reducing extent of expression of the Axis II disorder
   3. Especially in comorbid adjustment disorders, crisis-oriented psychotherapy, including supportive and cognitive-behavioral techniques, can help regain psychological homeostasis (using healthier defenses and minimizing less healthy or more destructive patterns)

E. If purely a problem of personality disorder, often these patients do not come into clinical contact for the problem unless external forces are involved; e.g., threats of divorce by spouse; child or adult protective services; family or criminal court systems.

F. Psychotherapy has the following features.
   1. Longer-term psychotherapy: indicated when disorders are severe enough to lead to behavioral sequelae that bring patients into frequent contact with acute mental health services (e.g., via recurrent suicide attempts)
   2. Psychotherapy of various lengths: for less severe disorders and when patients are self-referred to ameliorate what they perceive as dysfunctional patterns of behavior—a recognition that is prognostically a good sign

3. Techniques of psychotherapy vary considerably along supportive-expressive continuum based upon:
   a. Specific personality disorder
   b. Developmental phase
   c. Assessments of integrity of self
4. Research sparse on long-term outcome of psychotherapy for personalities (enormous number of difficult-to-quantify variables)
5. Longstanding clinical experience supports overall usefulness
   a. Parameters of optimal efficacy or cost-effectiveness not known
6. Dialectical Behavioral Therapy (DBT): an empirically-supported psychotherapy proven useful with borderline personality disorder (also used in bipolar disorder, binge eating disorder, and recurrent depression)
   a. Four modules in DBT group skills training
      i. *Core mindfulness skills* (becoming aware of emotions)
      ii. *Interpersonal effectiveness skills* (interpersonal skills training)
      iii. *Emotion modulation skills* (reducing or eliminating negative emotions)
      iv. *Distress tolerance skills* (learning to tolerate painful emotions)
G. Pharmacotherapy has the following features.
1. Has a place in some patients (especially in crisis)
2. Antipsychotics
   a. May be used to target transient psychotic or near-psychotic symptoms in patients with schizotypal, paranoid, or borderline personality disorders
   b. Short-term management of severe impulse or affect "dyscontrol" in severe cluster B disorders
3. Mood stabilizers (as lithium, carbamazepine, and valproate): may be helpful in longer run for the following
   a. Affective instability
   b. Impulsivity
   c. Anger attacks
4. Antidepressants: have utility
   a. Comorbid Axis I disorders
   b. Selective serotonin reuptake inhibitors—nonspecifically helpful in rage attacks (even in absence of depressive disorder)

5. Anxiolytics: usually for comorbid Axis I disorders
   a. Use benzodiazepines carefully.
      i. Chronic use may lead to disinhibited behaviors
      ii. High comorbidity with substance use disorders in personality disorders
   b. Buspirone: may be helpful in:
      i. Reduction of overall anxiety.
      ii. Reduction of rage attacks.

 MENTOR TIPS DIGEST

- The distinction between Axis II and I can be useful but sometimes arbitrary and difficult or impossible to make. For example, lifelong chronic depressive or anxiety symptoms become inseparably intertwined with personality. Therefore, it is important to accept this possible coexistence and treat symptomatic manifestations as best as possible.
- Beware of diagnosing or labeling patients with personality disorder *solely* on how they appear to you *now*. Dysfunctional patterns need to be enduring rather than artifacts of patients' current state.
- Given the disadvantages of DSM-IV-TR's categories of personality disorders, it is not surprising that clinicians need to use a variety of perspectives beyond DSM-ese to understand and work with patients with personality difficulties.
- A person with schizoid personality may later receive a diagnosis of schizophrenia if individual goes on to develop frank psychotic symptoms, but many persons have stable schizoid personalities throughout their lives without developing psychotic illness.
- Persons with paranoid personality disorder may be more likely than others to become flagrantly psychotic at times of stress; an additional diagnosis of appropriate psychotic disorder would be made.
- In working with patients with borderline personality disorder, considerable affect can often be evoked in caregivers. The caregiver must monitor this affect carefully to provide appropriate, professional, effective treatments.

- With more research, either avoidant personality disorder or social phobia may be eliminated from future DSMs.
- In obsessive-compulsive personality disorder, the term "obsessiveness" retains its familiar meaning from lay usage, different from the obsessions of obsessive-compulsive disorder. Keep in mind that some degree of obsessiveness is useful to completing tasks and achieving goals.
- Persons with passive-aggressive personality disorder control their lives and environment through inaction.
- In many quarters, treatment of personality disorders has a rather hopeless reputation. Empirical research has shown that personality usually remains remarkably stable throughout adulthood. Yet, being realistic about prognosis does not mean feeling hopeless.

Chapter Self-Test Questions

Circle the correct answer. After you have responded to the questions, check your answers in Appendix A.

1. A person's enduring patterns of thinking, feeling, acting, and reacting is referred to as:

   a. Affect.

   b. Conduct.

   c. Mood.

   d. Personality.

2. In DSM-IV-TR's multiaxial assessment scheme, personality disorder diagnoses should be written on:

   a. Axis I.

   b. Axis II.

   c. Axis III.

   d. Axis IV.

3. A 39-year-old woman is needy, clingy, dependent on others for support and reassurance but does not have these characteristics when not in

depressed periods of her recurrent major depression. Which of the following is (are) the patient's diagnosis (es)?

a. Dependent personality disorder

b. Major depression and avoidant personality disorder

c. Major depression and dependent personality disorder

d. Major depression, recurrent

4. When personality deviates markedly from cultural expectations, is inflexible and pervasive across a broad range of situations, and causes subjective distress or impairment in interpersonal relationships or other role functioning (e.g., work, school), this is referred to as a(n):

a. Adjustment disorder.

b. Anxiety disorder.

c. Personality disorder.

d. Personality trait.

5. The cluster of personality disorders that exhibit significant anxiety and fear, such as avoidant, dependent, and obsessive-compulsive disorder, are referred to in DSM-IV-TR as:

a. Cluster A.

b. Cluster B.

c. Cluster C.

d. Cluster D.

 See the testbank CD for more self-test questions.

OTHER PSYCHOPATHOLOGICAL CATEGORIES

Michael R. Privitera, MD, MS, and Jeffrey M. Lyness, MD

I. Medically Unexplained Symptoms

A. Overview

1. Patients frequently present (to physicians of all specialties) with physical symptoms that cannot be explained in kind or degree by identifiable physical pathology

2. Psychiatric disorders *may* or *may not* help explain patient's presentation

3. Medically unexplained symptoms (MUS) may mean:

   a. There is no objective evidence of identifiable cause or pathogenesis that could account for symptoms.

   b. Symptoms are out of proportion to what would usually be expected from any identified cause or pathogenesis.

4. Known physical disorders may be affected by emotional or psychological processes in various ways

   a. Anxiety contributing to symptoms of medical illness (e.g., gastrointestinal hypermobility or irritable bowel syndrome)

   b. Stress-induced worsening of primary medical conditions (e.g., angina, diabetic hyperglycemia, asthmatic bronchospasm)

   c. Health-related behaviors affecting medical course (e.g., lifestyle activities that are risks of onset or worsening of specific medical disorders)

5. Differential diagnosis

   a. "I do not know": important to be willing to admit ignorance

    i. Occult physical illness can later declare itself more definitively: follow-up studies on patients with "somatization" disorder show high rate of neurological and other conditions

    ii. Psychiatric disorder diagnosis depends both on *absence* of physical disorder and *presence* of specific clinical features consistent with psychiatric diagnosis

> Just because you do not know what the physical disorder is does not necessarily mean it must be "psychiatric." **XI 7**

    iii. Taking stance of ignorance may be useful in allying with patient and managing ongoing unexplainable symptoms (see discussion on treatment)

  b. Review possible illness perception-amplifying/generating disorders

    i. Depression: somatic symptoms or rumination about somatic issues may accompany major depression; successful treatment of depression may eliminate or greatly reduce patient's somatic concerns

    ii. Anxiety disorders: anxiety may be accompanied by wide range of somatic symptoms (e.g., panic disorder common cause of referrals to cardiologist for chest discomfort)

    iii. Delusions: somatic worry may reach delusional proportions and may occur in course of several psychiatric disorders (Schizophrenia, Schizoaffective Disorder, Delusional Disorder [primary or secondary], Mood Disorders, Dementia, and Delirium)

  c. Abnormal illness behaviors, such as Malingering, Factitious Disorder, and Somatoform Disorders (Table 14.1).

6. Assessment of MUS **XI 6**

  a. Be clear that patients' symptoms often cannot be adequately explained by objectively demonstrable disease (principle clear in theory, not always easy to put into operation).

  b. Considerable clinical judgment is required to determine extent of specialist consultation, laboratory test, or other procedures.

  c. Begin to explore patient's psychiatric symptoms and psychosocial context as *part of initial and ongoing evaluation.*

TABLE 14.1 Disorders Presenting as Medically Unexplained Symptoms [14]

Diagnosis	Major Characteristics	Production of Symptoms	Motivation for Production of Symptoms
Malingering	Lies for external goal: money, avoid undesired duty, obtain drugs	Conscious	Conscious
Factitious Disorder	Sole motivation of assuming sick role	Conscious	Unconscious
Somatoform Disorders			
Somatization Disorder	Numerous somatoform symptoms from multiple organ symptoms over many years	Unconscious	Unconscious
Undifferentiated Somatoform Disorder	One to multiple symptoms just shy of Somatization Disorder, ≥6 months in duration	Unconscious	Unconscious
Somatoform Disorder NOS	One to multiple symptoms just shy of Somatization Disorder, <6 months in duration	Unconscious	Unconscious
Conversion Disorder	Monosymptomatic—mimics neurological disease	Unconscious	Unconscious
Pain Disorder	Monosymptomatic—pain	Unconscious	Unconscious
Hypochondriasis	Undue worry about having a serious disease, based on misinterpretation of normal or abnormal bodily symptoms or functions	Unconscious	Unconscious
Body Dysmorphic Disorder	Preoccupied with imagined or greatly exaggerated defects in physical appearance	Unconscious	Unconscious

    i. Facilitates rapid and accurate assessment
    ii. Communicates that you consider emotional factors as seriously as physical factors
    iii. Too often, exploration of these dimensions deferred until numerous tests have failed to reveal clear physical etiology
  d. Learn whether patient has had any previous episodes of MUS.
  e. In psychiatric differential diagnosis:
    i. First delineate disorders with most specific treatments (Depression, Anxiety Disorders, and Psychosis)
      (1) If identified, education and discussion of treatment should begin *concomitant with* parallel physical workup
    ii. If these psychiatric conditions not present and still MUS
      (1) You probably have by now enough sense of psychosocial context to speculate about somatoform or factitious disorders and malingering.
      (2) You will also have begun to build alliance with the patient that will form basis of management.
B. Malingering
  1. *Not a mental disorder,* but is in medical differential diagnosis and listed in DSM-IV-TR
  2. Person consciously and intentionally produces false or grossly exaggerated physical or psychological symptoms—i.e., *lies*
  3. Some specific external goal in mind
    a. Obtaining money (e.g., lawsuits or workers compensation)
    b. Avoiding undesired duty (e.g., job, prison term)
    c. Obtaining drugs
  4. Should be suspected if:
    a. Strong external incentives favor symptom production
    b. Symptoms difficult to reconcile with objective findings
    c. Compliance with diagnostic or therapeutic recommendations is poor
    d. Person has other evidence for antisocial personality disorder
  5. Unless lie is directly exposed, can be difficult to diagnose malingering with certainty
C. Factitious Disorders
  1. Patient intentionally feigns or produces physical or psychological symptoms or signs *with sole motivation of assuming sick role* (other external motivations as in malingering are absent)

2. Physical symptom subtypes
   a. Common, nonperegrinating (not traveling), usually without aliases; sometimes still called Munchausen's syndrome
   b. Full-blown Munchausen's syndrome (travels hospital to hospital, city to city, state to state), often using aliases to conceal identity and avoid detection
3. Examples of sign production
   a. Placing drop of blood in one's urine leading to workup for hematuria
   b. Self-injecting foreign materials to produce low-grade fevers
   c. Self-injecting insulin to produce hypoglycemia
   d. Ingesting anticoagulants to produce bleeding
4. As a result, may undergo numerous invasive diagnostic or therapeutic procedures
5. Often history of employment in the health professions or other connection with them
6. Some adult patients produce symptoms in their children and seek pediatric attention: known as Munchausen's by proxy
7. Why people do this to assume sick role—speculations include:
   a. Desire to be taken care of
   b. Form close relationships with health-care providers
   c. Direct or displaced hostility toward health-care professionals ("tricking" them) or toward themselves (subjecting themselves to uncomfortable or dangerous procedures)
8. Optimal treatment

 Treatment for factitious disorder tends to be difficult, even for the few patients who allow psychiatric contact.

   a. Setting limits on symptom-producing behavior (via confrontation or behavioral therapies)
   b. Psychodynamic psychotherapies (address underlying character issues that led to need for seeking care or expressing rage in such dysfunctional fashion)
   c. Alerting nearby hospitals and emergency rooms (within bounds of law and ethics) to patient's presentation—goal of raising level of suspicion to reduce unnecessary tests, procedures, or surgeries

d. For Munchausen's by proxy, child protective laws allow safe-guarding of patients and may facilitate/demand psychiatric evaluation of parent/caregiver

D. Somatoform Disorders

1. Overview

   a. Several listed in DSM-IV-TR

   b. Commonality: have distressing symptoms that are either unrelated to or grossly in excess of what would be expected from identifiable medical conditions

   c. Symptoms are *not* consciously feigned or produced (patients are not malingering or have factitious disorder)

   d. Psychological factors generally presumed to be contributory to physical symptoms; motivation unconscious

2. Somatoform types

   a. Somatization Disorder (also known as Briquet's syndrome)

     i. Have numerous somatoform symptoms from multiple organ symptoms over many years

     ii. Chronic

     iii. More prevalent in women

     iv. Comorbidity with personality disorder and other Axis I disorders (e.g., commonly substance use, anxiety disorders) 🔲②

   b. Pain Disorder

     i. Monosymptomatic somatoform conditions, with predominant symptom being pain

   c. Conversion Disorder

     i. Usually monosymptomatic somatoform condition that mimics neurological disease; symptom is alteration in voluntary motor or sensory function; examples: conversion blindness, paralysis, or "nonelectrical" seizures

   d. Undifferentiated Somatoform Disorder

     i. Grab-bag category

     ii. Patients with somatoform symptoms that are *not*:

       (1) Predominantly pain or motor/sensory

       (2) Sufficient in number or duration to meet full-fledged somatization disorder

> Patients with Undifferentiated Somatoform Disorder range from one symptom to those with multiple symptoms just shy of Briquet's level

> presentation. Presentation needs to be at least 6 months long, otherwise falls into even more heterogeneous category Somatoform Disorder NOS.

  e. Hypochondriasis
   i. Not defined by symptom presentation
   ii. Undue worry about having serious disease, based on misinterpretation of normal or abnormal bodily symptoms or functions
   iii. Cannot be delusional proportions
   iv. Typically leads to frequent contact with medical or other professionals, whose reassurances fail to sufficiently assuage patient
  f. Body Dysmorphic Disorder
   i. Patient preoccupied with imagined or greatly exaggerated defects in physical appearance
   ii. May involve any body part
   iii. Examples: unrealistic worry about:
    (1) Thinning hair
    (2) Large or crooked nose
    (3) Genital size or appearance
   iv. Patient may seek physical remedies from dermatologist, plastic surgeon, other specialists

> Body Dysmorphic Disorder may be qualitatively distinct from other somatoform disorders. It might be related pathogenetically to obsessive-compulsive disorder, suggested by partial improvement with serotonin reuptake inhibitors.

  3. Interventions: matched to situation (Tables 14.2 and 14.3).

II. Other Psychopathological Categories
  A. Overview
   1. Brief tour through remaining categories of DSM-IV-TR
   2. Mastery of these (as a whole) less important for most trainees rotating through psychiatry first time, compared with other disorders already mentioned
   3. Developmental and child psychiatry disorders and psychiatric subspecialty areas discussed in Chapter 19

TABLE 14.2

General Management of Somatoform Disorders [XI 6]

What to Say Regarding:		
	Medically unexplained symptoms (MUS)	**Do not** tell patient: • "Nothing is wrong" • Somatic symptoms are "not real" • "All in your head" • "Due to" emotional problems (destroys alliance and is invalidating to patient's experience of distress) **Do:**
Cause of MUS		• Convey your understanding of patient's suffering • Confess your ignorance as to cause of symptoms • Offer reassurances: no evidence of life-threatening illness; no indications for further tests at this time (combined with validating and empathic comments underscoring patient's real distress)
Chances of improvement	If *no prior MUS* and *recent onset* of symptoms	• Offer encouragement of likelihood of spontaneous recovery in near future
	Chronic MUS	• Lower expectation that symptoms can be fixed in near future • Offer encouragement: patient may be able to function better (despite symptoms) by not allowing symptoms to dominate life

What to do Regarding:		
Levels of insight	*Open* to role of psychological or psychosocial factors	• Begin to explore issues in supportive psychotherapy • Referral to mental health specialists as indicated (and accepted by patient)
	Hostile to discussion of psychological issues	• Approach more obliquely: "Having this ongoing symptom must be distressing for you." (may take weeks, months, or never for psychological breakthrough) • Sometimes doing no harm is all you can do
Office visits		• See chronic MUS patients at regularly scheduled appointments (fosters alliance; may reduce unnecessary utilization of symptoms and health-care resources; to tell patient "come back if you need to" is an invitation for symptoms or disability to worsen)

TABLE 14.3	Management of Somatoform Disorders Matched to Specific Symptoms and Situations XI 6	
Symptom/Situation	**Management**
Physiological disturbance/emotional arousal	• Pharmacological and somatic treatments • Biofeedback • Relaxation training • Stress management
Attention to body	• Distraction • Attention refocus • Hypnosis
Attribution of sensations to illness Illness worry Catastrophizing Demoralization Communication of distress Help seeking	• Reattribution • Behavioral interventions • Psychoeducation • Reframing • Desensitization • Reassurance • Response prevention • Modification of illness behavior
Avoidance Disability Social response	• Exposure • Graded activity • Couple and family therapy • Support groups • Consultation to health-care providers • Intervention in compensation system

B. Eating Disorders XIII 1
   1. Abnormalities in eating behavior
   2. Two main types
      a. Anorexia Nervosa
        i. Fail to maintain a minimally normal weight for age and height
        ii. Some combination of limiting caloric intake, exercising to burn off calories, or purging activities (self-induced vomiting; misuse of laxatives, enemas, or diuretics)
        iii. Distorted sense of body weight, shape, or image

       (1) Fear of gaining weight even when dangerously underweight

    iv. Postmenarcheal girls also have amenorrhea

  b. Bulimia Nervosa

    i. Maintain adequate weight

    ii. Recurrent episodes of binge eating (discrete periods of large food intake along with sense of lack of control of intake)

    iii. Compensatory behaviors for binges to prevent weight gain (purging, fasting, or excessive exercise, laxatives, enemas, diuretics)

    iv. Distorted self-image of body or overall self-image excessively tied to perception of body shape or size

C. Dissociative Disorders `XII 2`

  1. Presence of dissociative symptoms

    a. Disruptions in otherwise normal-functioning consciousness, memory, identity, or environmental perception

  2. Symptoms may occur as part of other disorders (i.e., post-traumatic and acute stress disorders)

  3. Primary Dissociative Disorders

    a. Dissociative Amnesia

      i. One or more episodes of memory loss (often of stressful or traumatic events) that cannot be explained by physical or other mental disorder

    b. Dissociative Fugue

      i. Sudden and unexpected travel away from usual environments and either:

        (1) Assume new identity

        (2) Confused about past experiences and identity

    c. Dissociative Identity Disorder (formerly and still popularly known as Multiple Personality Disorder)

      i. Shifts among two or more distinct identities or personality states

      ii. Each has its own enduring patterns of thinking, feeling, and acting (think of popular media examples such as *Sybil* or *The Three Faces of Eve*)

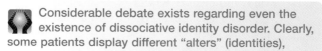

Considerable debate exists regarding even the existence of dissociative identity disorder. Clearly, some patients display different "alters" (identities),

> some in dramatic fashion. Whether these patients have psychopathology distinguishable from other mental disorders (e.g., borderline personality disorder) and how much the creation of alters depends upon the psychotherapist's expectations is quite controversial.

    d. Depersonalization Disorder
       i. Episodes of feeling physically and mentally detached from one's own mind and body
      ii. Depersonalization may be seen in other mental disorders, such as Acute Stress or Panic Disorder
    e. Dissociative Disorder NOS
       i. Term for even less well-defined, or more unusual, cases of dissociation, such as what used to be called "psychogenic unresponsiveness"
D. Paraphilias `XIV 6-7`
    1. Characterized by recurrent, intense, and distressing or impairing sexual fantasies, urges, or behaviors
    2. Typically involve nonhuman objects, or humiliation of oneself or one's partner
    3. Specific types
      a. Exhibitionalism: exposing one's genitals to strangers
      b. Fetishism: arousal from inanimate objects such as undergarments
      c. Frotteurism: touching or rubbing against nonconsenting persons
      d. Pedophilia: sexually arousing fantasies, urges, or actions involving prepubescent children
      e. Sexual masochism: arousal related to being beaten, humiliated, or otherwise suffering
      f. Sexual sadism: arousal related to similar suffering inflicted on others
      g. Transvestic fetishism: arousal involving cross-dressing
      h. Voyeurism: arousal involving watching naked, disrobing, or sexually active unsuspecting other persons
E. Sexual Dysfunctions `XIV 4-5`
    1. Impairments in sexual desire or in psychophysiology of sexual response cycle
    2. Lifelong or of more recent onset

3. Generalized or limited to specific situations
4. Causes
   a. Known physiological factors (e.g., secondary sexual dysfunctions due to general medical conditions or substance-induced syndromes)
   b. Psychological factors
   c. Both
5. Primary sexual dysfunctions organized partly on phase of sexual response cycle
   a. Sexual desire disorders: hypoactive sexual desire, sexual aversion disorder
   b. Disorders of sexual arousal: male erectile or female arousal disorders
   c. Orgasmic disorders: Trouble attaining orgasm (female or male) and premature ejaculation
   d. Sexual pain disorders: dyspareunia and vaginismus (considered mental disorders only if not due to medical illness)
F. Gender Identity Disorder XIV 9
   1. Characterized by pervasive cross-gender identification and discomfort with one's actual gender
   2. Not merely cross-dressing but strong desire to behave in stereotypic cross-gender manners or be other gender
   3. Some (particularly those with childhood onset) seek sex-reassignment surgery
G. Impulse Control Disorders
   1. Failure to resist an impulse, drive, or temptation to perform an act that is harmful to self or others
   2. Often preceded by a growing sense of tension or arousal and followed by pleasure or relief
   3. May or may not be guilt or regrets
   4. These diagnoses used only if poor impulse control not explained by another mental disorder (e.g., fire setting as part of psychotic disorder)
   5. Specific categories
      a. Kleptomania: recurrent senseless stealing of objects
      b. Pyromania: fire setting
      c. Pathological gambling: broadly analogous in clinical features to addiction, although physiological dependence is obviously lacking

    d. Trichotillomania: pulling one's hair; may have clinical or neurobiological overlap with Obsessive-Compulsive Disorder

    e. Intermittent Explosive Disorder: discrete episodes of aggressivity; however, considerable controversy whether this exists as discrete disorder separate from other psychopathology

H. Adjustment Disorders

  1. Manifested by clinically significant emotional or behavioral symptoms that occur in direct response to specific stressful events

  2. Symptoms must resolve in 6 months after resolution of stressor

  3. Various specifiers are given to describe nature of symptoms (e.g., adjustment disorders with depressed mood, with anxiety, with mixed anxiety and depressed mood, with disturbance of conduct, with mixed disturbance of emotions and conduct, and ubiquitous "unspecified")

> Adjustment disorder diagnosis is *not* given if symptoms meet criteria for another Axis I condition, as stressful events often precipitate other mental disorders. Thus, someone who develops six depressive symptoms for a 4-week period after being fired would be diagnosed with major depression, *not* with adjustment disorder.

I. Sleep Disorders

  1. Overview

    a. Sleep is more than just "absence of wakefulness"

    b. Complex phenomenon involving variety of neurological, systemic, and mental activities

    c. Divided into: XV 1

      i. Rapid eye movement (REM) sleep: state in which dreams occur

      ii. Non-REM sleep: numbered stages, based on sleep depth

    d. Altered sleep is common symptom

      i. Sole symptom or part of constellation of mental or physical findings

      ii. Caused by:

        (1) Primary Sleep Disorder

        (2) Neurological or systemic disease or drugs ("secondary" sleep disorders)

(3) Idiopathic Psychiatric Disorder (e.g., insomnia or hypersomnia of major depressions) **XV 4**

2. Classification of sleep disorders **XV 3**

   a. Overview: has been confusing because DSM-IV-TR diagnoses have not always matched schemata proposed by others in the field

   b. Insomnias

      i. Difficulty initiating or maintaining sleep, or as nonrestorative (i.e., unrestful) sleep

      ii. Classified

        (1) Primary (idiopathic)

        (2) Secondary (e.g., due to psychiatric disorders, drugs, physical conditions)

   c. Hypersomnias

      i. Excessive sleepiness, whether manifested by lengthy "sleep episodes" (nighttime for most people) or daytime sleepiness

      ii. Classified: primary or secondary

   d. Dyssomnias (i.e., other difficulties with sleep)

      i. Narcolepsy

        (1) Irresistible attacks of refreshing daytime sleepiness

        (2) Cataplexy (brief episodes of sudden skeletal muscle atony)

        (3) Intrusion of REM sleep into wakeful-sleep interface, evidenced by hypnagogical (going to sleep) or hypnopompic (waking from sleep) hallucinations, or sleep paralysis while falling asleep or just awakening

      ii. Breathing-related sleep disorders

        (1) Caused by ventilatory abnormalities that disrupt sleep—leads to complaints of insomnia, daytime sleepiness, or both, including:

          (A) Obstructive sleep apnea: upper airway obstruction occurs during sleep

          (B) Central sleep apnea: cessation of ventilation without obstruction, presumed due to central nervous system factors

          (C) Central alveolar hypoventilation: alveolar hypoventilation, such as due to cor pulmonale, which is worsened during sleep

(D) Circadian rhythm sleep disorder: sleep disruption caused by mismatch between endogenous circadian rhythms and environmental cues or demands (e.g., "jet lag," sleep disorders in shift workers moving between night and day shift)

e. Parasomnias

   i. Defined as abnormal behavioral or physiological events during sleep, specific sleep stages, or transitions between waking and sleeping

     (1) Nightmares: recurrent and stressing or impairing bad dreams

     (2) Sleep terrors

        (A) Recurrent abrupt awakenings with autonomic and often affective suggestions of "terror"

        (B) No dream is recalled

        (C) Later, there is amnesia for whole episode

     (3) Sleepwalking: close to what is portrayed in movies, but individual does not perform terribly complex tasks [e.g., murders] while sleepwalking

MENTOR TIPS DIGEST

- Just because you do not know what the physical disorder is does not necessarily mean it must be "psychiatric." [XI 7]
- Treatment for Factitious Disorder tends to be difficult, even for the few patients who allow psychiatric contact.
- Patients with Undifferentiated Somatoform Disorder range from one symptom to those with multiple symptoms just shy of Briquet's level presentation. Presentation needs to be at least 6 months long, otherwise falls into even more heterogeneous category Somatoform Disorder NOS.

- Body Dysmorphic Disorder may be qualitatively distinct from other somatoform disorders. It might be related pathogenetically to Obsessive-Compulsive Disorder, suggested by partial improvement with serotonin reuptake inhibitors.
- Considerable debate exists regarding even the existence of Dissociative Identity Disorder. Clearly, some patients display different "alters" (identities), some in dramatic fashion. Whether these patients have psychopathology distinguishable from other mental disorders (e.g., Borderline Personality Disorder) and how much the creation of alters depends upon the psychotherapist's expectations is quite controversial.
- Adjustment disorder diagnosis is *not* given if symptoms meet criteria for another Axis I condition, as stressful events often precipitate other mental disorders. Thus, someone who develops six depressive symptoms for a 4-week period after being fired would be diagnosed with major depression, *not* with adjustment disorder.

Resources

Epstein RM, Quill TE, McWhinney IR: Somatization reconsidered. Archives of Internal Medicine 150:215–222, 1999.

Looper KJ, Kirmayer LJ: Behavioral medicine approaches to somatoform disorders. Journal of Consulting and Clinical Psychology 70:810–827, 2002.

Seaburn DB, et al: Physician responses to ambiguous patient symptoms. Journal of General Internal Medicine 20:525–530, 2005.

Chapter Self-Test Questions

Circle the correct answer. After you have responded to the questions, check your answers in Appendix A.

1. Known physical disorders may be affected by emotional or psychological processes in various ways. Which of the following is an example of a condition where anxiety directly contributes to the production of the symptoms?

    a. Acute appendicitis

    b. Gastric carcinoma

    c. Irritable bowel syndrome

    d. Osteoarthritis

2. Known physical disorders may be affected by emotional or psychological processes in various ways. Which of the following is an example of a condition where psychological stress induces a significant worsening of the primary symptoms of the medical condition?

    a. Asthmatic bronchospasm

    b. Hypokalemia

    c. Pancreatic carcinoma

    d. Tibia fracture

3. In working with patients who have medically unexplained symptoms, it is important to be able to admit our ignorance about the cause of the symptoms. Which of the following is a significant reason that it is important to do so?

    a. Helps distinguish whether symptoms are feigned

    b. Helps many patients spontaneously recover

    c. It allows more testing paid for by the insurance company

    d. Occult physical illness may later declare itself more definitively

4. Which of the following is a common cause of referrals to a cardiologist for chest discomfort?

    a. Adjustment disorder with disturbance of conduct

    b. Manic episode

    c. Panic Disorder

    d. Schizophrenia

5. In evaluating a patient with unexplained physical symptoms of severe abdominal pain, you have also identified that the patient also has symptoms of a major depression. Which of the following would be the best approach in the care of this patient?

a. Education and discussion of treatment of major depression should begin *concomitant with* parallel physical workup.

b. Just work up the abdominal pain.

c. Reassure the patient that the abdominal pain and his depression should spontaneously get better.

d. Treat just the major depression and no physical workup.

See the testbank CD for more self-test questions.

PSYCHIATRIC
TREATMENTS

15

PSYCHOTHERAPIES

**Michael R. Privitera, MD, MS, and
Jeffrey M. Lyness, MD**

I. Overview

A. Narrow and most common use of term "psychotherapy" refers to a well-defined form of treatment

B. Broad sense of "psychotherapy" refers to beneficial effects for patient of relationship with physician or other health-care provider (XXI 1)

    1. Therefore, all clinicians use "psychotherapy" but neither they nor patients usually call it such

    2. All treatments and other interventions (medications, diagnostic interventions, surgery) depend on and occur within doctor-patient alliance

    3. Maintaining strong, positive therapeutic alliance must be goal for *all clinicians*, regardless of specialty

C. Several aspects of positive alliance are therapeutic (i.e., they help patient feel better)

D. Therapeutic factors in doctor-patient relationship may include:
  1. Empathy
    a. Patients feel better when they feel emotionally connected to a physician.
    b. "Connected to" includes feeling of being understood and a sense of being cared about and for (all implied in the term "empathy").
    c. A number of techniques in interviewing can communicate empathy (learned in coursework on basic interviewing skills).
  2. Role modeling
    a. Patients can feel reassured, calmed, or otherwise soothed by example of physician's demeanor (assuming enough alliance is present for example to be meaningful to patient)
    b. Examples
      i. If sufficient alliance:
        (1) Physician's attitude of realistic hopefulness may engender sense of hope in patient
        (2) Physician's expressed concern about a problem may lead to improved patient compliance with recommended interventions
      ii. If insufficient alliance:
        (1) Physician calm but gives impression of lack of concern for patient—patient unlikely to be reassured by physician's calmness
  3. Direct reassurance
    a. Often physicians must reassure patients by words as well as by demeanor
    b. Critical to maintain empathy while doing so
      i. Ensure that telling patient that symptom is not serious does not convey a sense of derision or condescension about patient's worry
      ii. Important interview skill is ability to communicate that you take patient's *concern* seriously although *symptom* does not worry you
  4. Education
    a. Basic task as physician: tell patient what you think
      i. How you understand what problem patient has
      ii. Why you are recommending your approach
    b. Nuances of task
      i. Variations in vocabulary, language style

    ii. *What* (i.e., how much) to say

    iii. *When* (i.e., timing)

    iv. *Who* (deciding whether or when to include family members or others in discussions)

  c. Useful technique for two broad reasons

    i. *Content* communicated: enables (and empowers) patients to know enough to join with you in making needed decisions

    ii. *Process* of education (if done properly): fosters both empathy and role modeling—expressing in action (if not words) your belief that the two of you are working together to address patient's concerns

5. Acknowledging ignorance

  a. Often you may be uncertain about diagnosis, prognosis, or other issues. Be explicit and clear with your patient about what you do and do not know.

  b. Convey how important or possible attaining such certainty is, and what you suggest to arrive at that needed clarity.

6. Recommendations

  a. Every patient contact should include some component of recommendations.

  b. Many times recommendations may be to do nothing or to continue the present course.

    i. Even in these situations making this explicit to patient:

      (1) Can be enormously reassuring to patient.

      (2) Helps ensure that nothing different is done.

    ii. May be while awaiting results of procedure or observing symptoms over time

  c. Recommendations often have two or more major components.

    i. What you anticipate will happen if treatment goes as expected: "Odds are good that your symptoms will gradually resolve over next 1–2 weeks, in which case continue the treatments you are using."

    ii. What to do if treatment does not go as expected: "If symptoms do not improve or you develop fever, call me and we will need to reevaluate at that time." (Note how education and recommendations coexist in this statement.)

  d. Careful attention to maintaining treatment alliance by use of education, empathy, and other factors mentioned above will maximize the likelihood that your patient will follow your recommendations, or if the patient chooses not to, the situation can be openly discussed (finding alternatives and maintaining healthy alliance). **XXI 5**

 Being conscious of aspects of positive alliance with patients will help you refine your interpersonal techniques to foster development and maintenance of positive alliances.

E. Formal psychotherapy versus informal "psychotherapy" (non-psychotherapy doctor-patient encounters)
  1. Formal psychotherapy: explicit acknowledgement and education (by referral process) that talking itself is intended to be therapeutic; flows naturally from explanation of treatment goals and methods
    a. Goals usually involve amelioration of troublesome feelings or patterns of actions.
  2. Informal "psychotherapy": therapeutic value of alliance is left unspoken or implied or obliquely referred to as doctor's "bedside manner"
F. Remainder of chapter surveys some of most common (formal) psychotherapy styles and their clinical applications

II. The Supportive-Expressive Continuum XXI 1
A. Overview
  1. These approaches are psychodynamic psychotherapies, based on psychodynamic principles (briefly discussed in Chapter 2)
  2. Two broad types: *supportive* and *expressive*
  3. Are convenient way to convey differing essences of approaches
    a. Skilled psychodynamic psychotherapist must be flexible, not limited by arbitrary boundaries
  4. Useful to consider supportive and expressive psychotherapies as two ends of a *spectrum* of psychodynamic psychotherapy
  5. Therapist must choose where to be on spectrum at any given time with particular patient
    a. Some at one end of spectrum
    b. Some are admixture of supportive and expressive techniques
    c. Some may shift during therapy
      i. Supportive during crises or symptom exacerbation

     ii. Expressive during relative stability or after period of supportive approach

> In thinking about psychotherapy, keep a sense of flexibility in mind. In practice many therapists usefully employ a mixture of psychodynamic, behavioral, and cognitive approaches as well as a mixture of individual, family, and group modalities.

B. Supportive psychotherapy

  1. Therapist formulates patient in psychodynamic terms (as one part of overall psychiatric formulation)

  2. Problematic conscious intrapsychic and interpersonal patterns identified (in collaboration with patient)

    a. Using this framework identifies goals for psychotherapy

  3. Most prominent techniques employed: nonspecific skills that have been previously mentioned in doctor-patient relationship

    a. Empathic listening

    b. Role modeling

    c. Education

    d. Recommendations

  4. All in service of:

    a. Maintaining positive therapeutic alliance

    b. Achieving patient-specific goals

  5. Given definition of psychotherapy, might seem like physician is simply "being there," as if anyone could accomplish this task

    a. Takes great skill to maintain positive alliance with many patients (e.g., when angry, withdrawn, "acting out" by noncompliance, or other self-destructive behaviors during therapy)

    b. Uses psychodynamic understanding of patient to shape response to such disruptions in alliance

    c. Although notions of unconscious (including transference and earlier developmental events' effect on current behaviors) are crucial to formulations, only rarely are direct interpretations of these processes offered to patient

    d. Most therapist comments take form of:

      i. Questioning

      ii. Clarifications

  iii. Confrontations (regarding overtly manifest thoughts and
    behaviors)
  iv. Suggestions

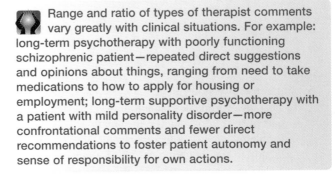

    Range and ratio of types of therapist comments
    vary greatly with clinical situations. For example:
long-term psychotherapy with poorly functioning
schizophrenic patient—repeated direct suggestions
and opinions about things, ranging from need to take
medications to how to apply for housing or
employment; long-term supportive psychotherapy with
a patient with mild personality disorder—more
confrontational comments and fewer direct
recommendations to foster patient autonomy and
sense of responsibility for own actions.

  6. Table 15.1 basic guide to indications for supportive psychotherapy
C. Expressive psychotherapy
  1. Often referred to as "insight-oriented" therapy
  2. Like supportive therapy, also based on psychodynamic theories
  3. Techniques closer to those of traditional psychoanalysis
    (discussed in next section)
  4. Specifically, direct suggestions or recommendations to patient
    are kept minimum
  5. Emphasis on interpretations of behavior, related to:
    a. Current unconscious mental processes
    b. Developmental issues and relationship to current mental func-
      tioning
    c. Direct interpretations of transference, particularly negative
      transference
    d. Interpretations lead to *insight*
      i. Patient comes to understand both *what* and *why* of trouble-
        some thoughts, feelings, and actions (which helps to make
        needed changes).
      ii. Obtaining such insight is not easy.
      iii. Unconscious mental processes are unconscious for a reason.
        (1) *Resistance* to interpretations may be demonstrated by
          patient
    e. Successful expressive therapy depends on positive transference
      (therapeutic alliance directly analogous to that of supportive

TABLE 15.1		
Indications for Supportive Psychotherapy XXI 1		
Indication	Comments	Goals
Crisis	Time of symptomatic exacerbation or regressed functions in patients with wide variety of psychiatric disorders	• Help patient regain psychic equilibrium
Long-term therapy with severely ill	Patients with chronic mental illness, particularly psychotic disorders; more severe variants of mood or personality disorders, may become worse with attempts at expressive psychotherapy; typically used in combination with medications or psychosocial interventions (e.g., case management, enriched housing, day programs)	• Psychoeducation • Treatment compliance • Successful negotiation through stressful events • Progress toward other specified goals (e.g., obtaining or maintaining a job, developing more friends or other social supports)
Other settings	Used in clinical settings not covered by above categories when • Specific goals exist for treatment with psychotherapy • No indications for behavioral, cognitive, or other specific psychotherapies • Expressive psychotherapy unlikely to be effective or tolerated	• Specific to situation

psychotherapy and any doctor-patient relationship), which provides framework for working through any resistance

f. Sessions are usually held at least weekly, sometimes two to three times a week, either to:

   i. Help manage crises or symptomatic exacerbations (in which case temporarily more towards supportive end of continuum)

   ii. Help overcome resistance and otherwise accelerate pace of insight and clinical improvement

6. Tailor treatment depending on situation

> Remember that patients need to be well enough to tolerate certain forms of expressive psychotherapy. For example, if a patient is admitted for suicidal ideation in Major Depression, and you discover the patient has a history of sexual abuse, do not delve into the details involved in the abuse or the feelings engendered. Patient's defenses would not be strong enough to deal with such highly charged memories while depressed and would likely make the depression and suicidal ideation worse, extending the illness.

7. Table 15.2 is a basic guide to indications for expressive psychotherapy.

III. Psychoanalysis

A. "Pure" psychoanalysis comprises small percentage of psychotherapies in broad spectrum of clinical practices.

B. Psychoanalysts may be psychiatrists, psychologists, or "lay analysts."

   1. All have undergone extensive training at psychoanalytic institutes.

C. Psychoanalysis involves 4- or 5-hour–long sessions per week, typically extending for several years.

D. Patient encouraged to express freely all thoughts and associations that come to mind during sessions.

   1. To facilitate this process and maximize intensity of transference reactions, patient reclines on couch while therapist sits out of patient's visual field.

   2. Analyst makes extensive use of interpretations.

      a. In "here and now" (e.g., transference interpretations)

      b. As related to developmental issues and earlier life events

TABLE 15.2

Indications for Expressive Psychotherapy (XXI 1)

Situations		Comments
Conditions	Relatively mild personality disorders (or personality-related difficulties)	Used to treat symptoms or aid "personal growth"
	Less severe Axis I conditions (such as mild mood or anxiety disorders)	Especially when superimposed on personality difficulties
Clinical characteristics (their absence suggests patient will not benefit from or tolerate such treatment)	Motivation for change	Self-evident
	Psychological mindedness	Ability to observe one's own internal state (introspection) and make sense of personal observations in psychological terms
	Ability to form a therapeutic alliance	Demonstrated by previous successful intimate relationships, capacity to tolerate one's own negative affects, and reasonable amount of impulse control

*Goals for all: *insight* necessary for needed changes.

E. Psychoanalysis is an extremely intensified version of expressive psychotherapy. (Historically, the reverse is true: face-to-face expressive psychotherapy evolved as less intense version of psychoanalysis, which is more suitable for sicker patients.)

F. Psychoanalysis is intended to address longstanding unconscious conflicts and personality issues.

   1. Symptomatic relief is expected by-product of this process eventually, but not a short-term goal

      a. *Not suitable for most acute Axis I disorders.*

G. Other factors limit the usefulness of psychoanalysis.

   1. Expense considerable, largely or entirely out of pocket

   2. Patients with moderate to severe personality disorders or with diathesis toward psychosis: unlikely to tolerate strong transference reactions that emerge from analysis

   3. Most persons who undergo psychoanalysis relatively healthy, with at most mild personality troubles or neurotic symptoms such as mild depression and anxiety

   4. Most analytic patients have high motivation for change and for exploration of internal self

IV. Brief Psychodynamic Psychotherapy

A. Supportive-expressive psychotherapy often used successfully for brief course (e.g., 2 or 3 months)

B. Following circumstances often apply

   1. Discrete focal problem can be identified.

      a. Should be of recent onset or exacerbation

      b. Often a response to a recent stressor

      c. May manifest as:

         i. Intrapsychic symptoms

         ii. Interpersonal discord

         iii. Decline from baseline level of functioning in one or several life roles

   2. Patient must be motivated to use psychotherapy.

   3. An explicit "treatment contract" is reached with the patient.

      a. Set frequency of visits

      b. Total duration of sessions

      c. Patient and therapist agree to work on focal problem

   4. It is explicitly recognized that longer-term psychological issues may influence the focal problem.

      a. Areas for benefit from longer-term psychotherapy only identified, as treatment entirely focused on issues directly related to focal problem

   5. The therapist must decide (in assessment or early treatment phase) how much to use *interpretations* (almost solely of the

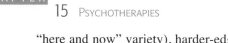

"here and now" variety), harder-edged *confrontations,* or *clarifications* and *guidance/recommendations* (see indications for supportive-expressive therapy that are used to inform this decision).

V. Behavioral and Cognitive Psychotherapy

A. As mentioned in Chapter 2, *behavioral* approaches to psychotherapy are rooted in learning theory.
1. Reinforcement: used to promote desirable behaviors and reduce undesirable ones
2. Patients learn:
   a. Can endure feelings or circumstances they previously thought unendurable
   b. Can get emotional needs met without resorting to troublesome, undesired behavior
3. Learning occurs through series of mental or action-oriented exercises, in therapy sessions and homework assignments between sessions

B. *Cognitive* therapy helps patients alter dysfunctional patterns of thinking.
1. Is rooted in cognitive psychology (way people think affects way people feel)
2. Through psychoeducation and specific assignments (in session and between sessions) patients identify cognitive distortions and replace them with more flexible thoughts that do not lead directly to undesired symptoms

 In some ways cognitive therapy is a behavioral approach to thoughts rather than external actions.

C. Cognitive and behavioral approaches are often combined in clinical practice (hence, the commonly used term "cognitive behavioral therapy" [CBT]).

D. Therapists take an active approach in administering CBT.
1. Must offer considerable psychoeducation, reassurance, and positive expectations to maximize likelihood of patient compliance with specific assignments and tasks
2. Efficacy results from particular techniques, but overall effectiveness depends on positive treatment alliance

BOX 15.1

Clinical Circumstances Useful for Cognitive Behavioral Therapy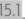

- Specific phobias (as primary treatment)
- Most other anxiety disorders (primary, co-primary, or adjunctive treatment)
- Anxiety symptoms as part of other psychiatric disorders
- Eating disorders
- Sexual dysfunctions
- Depressive syndromes
- Substance use disorders
- Specific problematic cognitions or behaviors (e.g., suicidality, self-mutilation, aggressive outbursts) as part of variety of organic mental syndromes including developmental disorders, (e.g., autism), mental retardation, dementias, or other secondary syndromes
- Specific problematic cognitions or behaviors seen as part of variety of idiopathic mental syndromes, including schizophrenia and personality disorders
- Variety of psychosomatic (or psychophysiological) disorders in which relaxation techniques or biofeedback may be useful, such as chronic headache or other pain syndromes, hypertension, and irritable bowel syndrome

E. Cognitive, behavioral, and cognitive behavioral therapies are useful in a broad range of clinical circumstances (Box 15.1).

VI. Dialectical Behavioral Therapy (DBT)
A. Overview
1. Based on a biosocial theory of Borderline Personality Disorder (BPD), now also being used in Bipolar Disorder, Binge-Eating Disorder, and recurrent depression
   a. Emotionally vulnerable individual growing up within a particular set of *environmental circumstances:* invalidating environment
   b. "Emotionally vulnerable": autonomic nervous system reacts excessively to low levels of stress and takes longer than normal to return to baseline
      i. As a child, behaviors oscillate between opposite poles of emotional inhibition, attempting to gain acceptance;

combining with invalidating environment to produce symptoms of BPD
  ii. "Dialectical" (classical philosophy): form of argument in which, first, assertion made ("thesis"), second, opposing formulation made ("antithesis"), finally, "synthesis" sought between two positions
  iii. Key dialectic: *acceptance* on one hand and *change* on other
  iv. Theory not yet supported by direct empirical evidence, but clinical efficacy of DBT does have substantial empirical support
B. DBT treatment
  1. Therapy is behavioral, as focuses on behaviors and current factors leading to behaviors
  2. Primary modes of therapy include:
    a. Individual therapy
      i. Uses a hierarchy such as decreasing suicidal behaviors, therapy-interfering behaviors, those that interfere with quality of life, and other behaviors
    b. Group skills training
      i. Core mindfulness skills (becoming aware of emotions)
      ii. Interpersonal effectiveness skills (interpersonal skills training)
      iii. Emotion modulation skills (reducing or eliminating negative emotions)
      iv. Distress tolerance skills (learn to tolerate painful emotions)
    c. Telephone contact
      i. However therapist has right to set clear limits
    d. Therapist consultation
      i. Working together with other therapists, may include therapist support and training

VII. Group Psychotherapy
A. Variety of groups available to patients
B. Use therapeutic leverage of group process
  1. Sense of belonging to group, gaining support from one's peers, and (in some groups) being confronted by one's peers can be enormously powerful in helping effect desired changes.

C. Groups may differ greatly along several dimensions
1. Group leadership
   a. Self-help groups
   b. Groups led by professionals of varied backgrounds, including (but not always limited to) psychotherapists
2. Meeting times
   a. Group sessions may be 30 minutes to 8 hours (60 to 90 minutes most common length; day-long sessions typically reserved for special workshops)
   b. Most meet weekly, but can be more or less often
3. Duration
   a. Pre-established number of sessions or weeks
   b. May exist indefinitely
4. Open or closed
   a. Open: accepting new members during group's existence
   b. Closed: not accepting new members after forming
   c. Some members may leave during group's existence; others expect membership to remain stable
5. Size
   a. Depends on group's theoretical orientation and treatment goals
   b. Most professionally led psychotherapy groups technically known as *small groups*
      i. Large enough to have true group dynamics (≥ 3 to 4 members), but small enough so each participant can maintain eye contact with all other participants (≤ 12 members)
6. Setting and context
   a. May serve outpatients; day or partial hospital patients; inpatients from psychiatric, rehabilitation, or other medical settings
   b. May serve residents of a group home, nursing home, or other residential facility
   c. May be a patient's sole treatment, or used in combination with other groups *(group program)* or other treatment modalities
7. Homogeneous versus heterogeneous patient population
   a. Some select patients based on common symptom, diagnosis, or demographic variable

  b. Other groups (like inpatient groups) take all comers

  c. Each type has own leverages and disadvantages

 8. Theoretical orientations

  a. May draw on any of many perspectives discussed for individual psychotherapies

  b. Most self-help groups are supportive, although may rely heavily on confrontation (e.g., Alcoholics Anonymous)

  c. Many professionally led

   i. Based on supportive-expressive psychodynamic techniques (with awareness of interpersonal dynamics within group as whole and intrapsychic dynamics of each member)

   ii. Cognitive-behavioral approaches, using group dynamics to support psychoeducation, and cognitive or behavioral assessments critical to these therapies (more likely to be diagnostically homogeneous so each member working on similar assignments aimed at changing similar behaviors)

   iii. Activities therapy groups

    (1) Range from task-oriented (e.g., arts and crafts) to process and interpersonally oriented therapy groups using music, art, or other modalities

 9. Goals

  a. Highly specific (e.g., maintaining alcohol sobriety, decreasing frequency of obsessions or compulsions)

  b. Broad (e.g., coping with chronic medical illness, fostering personal growth and maturation)

VIII. Family Therapy

A. Theoretically based on family systems perspectives

B. In practice, conducting family therapy resembles conducting group therapy, particularly how therapist integrates consideration of each member as an individual with recognition of dynamics among members (including dyads, triangles, and whole family)

C. Unlike group therapy: the family is a group with a long and complex history that predates contact with therapist, and most interactions within "group" (family) occur outside of therapy sessions

D. Therapist must understand traditions and styles of each family

E. Therapist must eventually be perceived by family as (almost) one of them, rather than as outsider

F. Families often enter therapy with one "identified patient" (IP) among them, i.e., one particular member most overtly symptomatic

   1. Recognition of IP as "one with problem" may be helpful or unhelpful for person and rest of family

   2. IP may be most severely disordered member, but dynamics of family interactions may perpetuate or exacerbate IP's symptoms

      a. Addressing these interactions offers one route to reducing symptoms and improving overall course of illness.

G. May use variety of techniques, including supportive, expressive, and cognitive-behavioral

   1. Barriers among these perspectives may be even less rigid than in other modalities.

H. Indications

   1. Not limited to specific diagnoses

   2. Whatever diagnosis of IP, clinical assessment of *family* leads to recommendation for family work

I. May be primary or adjunctive treatment

J. Often crucial in working with children, adolescents, and geriatric patients—necessitating close ties to family members around illness-related symptoms or treatment

   1. Given nature of disorders seen in these age groups

   2. Developmental issues common at these ages

K. Research demonstrates effectiveness of family therapy

   1. Using psychoeducation and supportive family therapy to reduce "expressed emotion" (openly expressed hostility or criticism) in order to reduce relapse in patients with schizophrenia or mood disorders

L. Couples therapy

   1. Variant of family therapy

   2. Essentially straightforward, psychodynamically informed psychotherapy applied to a dyadic relationship

   3. Sometimes more limited in focus and technique, such as behavioral approaches to sexual dysfunctions (sex therapy) with a couple

   4. Flexible in tailoring therapy to patient's (or couple's) needs

MENTOR TIPS DIGEST

- Being conscious of aspects of positive alliance with patients will help you refine your interpersonal techniques to foster development and maintenance of positive alliances.
- In thinking about psychotherapy, keep a sense of flexibility in mind. In practice many therapists usefully employ a mixture of psychodynamic, behavioral, and cognitive approaches as well as a mixture of individual, family, and group modalities.
- Range and ratio of types of therapist comments vary greatly with clinical situations. For example: long-term psychotherapy with poorly functioning schizophrenic patient—repeated direct suggestions and opinions about things, ranging from need to take medications to how to apply for housing or employment; long-term supportive psychotherapy with a patient with mild personality disorder—more confrontational comments and fewer direct recommendations to foster patient autonomy and sense of responsibility for own actions.
- Remember that patients need to be well enough to tolerate certain forms of expressive psychotherapy. For example, if a patient is admitted for suicidal ideation in Major Depression, and you discover the patient has a history of sexual abuse, do not delve into the details involved in the abuse or the feelings engendered. Patient's defenses would not be strong enough to deal with such highly charged memories while depressed and would likely make the depression and suicidal ideation worse, extending the illness.
- In some ways cognitive therapy is a behavioral approach to thoughts rather than external actions.

Resources

Linehan MM. Cognitive behavioral treatment of borderline personality disorder. The Guilford Press, New York and London, 1993.

Chapter Self-Test Questions

Circle the correct answer. After you have responded to the questions, check your answers in Appendix A.

1. Which of the following therapeutic factors in the doctor-patient relationship most directly conveys a feeling of being understood?

   a. Direct reassurance

   b. Education

   c. Empathy

   d. Role modeling

2. In the setting of sufficient alliance in the doctor-patient relationship, calm demeanor by the physician that helps instill calmness in the patient is referred to as:

   a. Direct reassurance.

   b. Education.

   c. Empathy.

   d. Role modeling.

3. You told your patient: "If symptoms do not improve or you develop fever, call me and we will reevaluate at that time." Which of the following therapeutic factors in the doctor-patient relationship were involved in this statement beside recommendation?

   a. Direct reassurance

   b. Education

   c. Empathy

   d. Role modeling

4. The form of psychotherapy that *all* physicians do in the setting of a positive doctor-patient alliance is often obliquely referred to as:

   a. Bedside manner.

   b. Cognitive-behavioral psychotherapy.

   c. Expressive psychotherapy.

   d. Psychoanalysis.

5. A 32-year-old-female, 6 weeks postpartum to the delivery of a healthy female baby and has no previous psychiatric history, was admitted for Major Depression with psychotic features. In the workup, you learn from her husband that she has a history of being sexually abused by her father when she was 12 years old. Which of the following would be *least* helpful to this patient in assisting her acute recovery?

a. Beginning antidepressants

b. Beginning antipsychotics

c. Exploration of her sexual abuse history

d. Supportive psychotherapy around activities of daily living.

 See the testbank CD for more self-test questions.

16

PHARMACOTHERAPY

Michael R. Privitera, MD, MS, and Jeffrey M. Lyness, MD

I. General Guidelines

A. Begin with most accurate diagnosis possible.
  1. Diagnosis will drive whether, when, what, and how drugs should be used.
B. Identify target symptoms for treatment.
  1. Documenting target symptoms and their severity allows you to more accurately monitor response.
C. Obtain detailed drug history of patient (and family history of response if similar disorder being treated).
  1. Drugs previously tried, dosage, duration, tolerability, side effects and response, reason for discontinuation
  2. If close relative had excellent response to fluoxetine, this may factor into your choice of antidepressant (i.e., pharmacogenetics of drug response)
D. An emergency should be the only exception to the above.
  1. Carefully think through (and document) rationale for all drug changes.
E. As best as clinical situations permits, change one variable at a time.
  1. Often pharmacotherapy, psychotherapy, and social treatments are started at the same time. Try not to add to the confusion by making more medication changes than necessary.
F. Evaluate response and side-effects and course of treatment.
  1. Evaluate
    a. Target symptoms and response
    b. Fluctuation in course
    c. Overall pattern of response

G. Consider cross-taper as a means of beginning a new drug from an old drug (as long as there are no drug-drug contraindications).
  1. Add new drug to old; see if significant side effects before beginning to taper off the old; helps differentiate new drug side effects from old drug withdrawal; may also prevent patients from "losing ground" they may have partially gained on old drug
H. When selecting *within* a drug class, consider:
  1. Side-effect burden risk in your particular patient.
    a. Is the person more likely to have side effects with one drug over another given age, comorbid medical problems, co-prescribed medications, etc?
  2. Drug-drug interaction possibilities.
    a. Pharmacodynamic and pharmacokinetic
  3. Cost.
    a. Many insurance companies now insist on generic failure(s) before brand names are allowed.
    b. Out-of-pocket costs to patient (which affects compliance) may vary depending on drug chosen or insurance plan of patient.
      i. For example, many indigent patients on government insurance (Medicaid) have little/no out-of-pocket costs, whereas other patients on private insurances may have significant co-pays.
    c. Generics should be considered if appropriate.
  4. Diagnostic subtype and likelihood of response.
    a. For example, severe major depression with melancholia may respond better to tricyclic, escitalopram, or serotonin/ norepinephrine reuptake inhibitors (SNRIs) than to most selective serotonin reuptake inhibitors (SSRIs)
  5. Patient preference.
    a. Some patients feel more confident in one drug than another, depending on what they have heard about the drug from Internet, friends, and media.
I. Keep in mind acute benefits versus long-term benefits and side effects in selecting drugs for a chronic condition.
  1. A drug might be considered in the acute situation (if reasonably effective) because it would be less troublesome to the patient for long-term use.

J. Rules of drug non-specificity are as follows.
  1. Drugs do not treat just one symptom or disorder.
    a. For example, antidepressants may be used to treat depressive symptoms, panic attacks, social phobia, obsessions or compulsions, primary insomnia, and enuresis.
  2. Drugs treat symptoms across diagnoses.
    a. Antidepressants treat depressive symptoms in major depression, bipolar disorder, depression secondary to Alzheimer's disease, and other disorders.
    b. Antipsychotics treat psychotic symptoms due to schizophrenia, delusional disorder, delirium, and other disorders.
  3. Drugs treat symptoms, not diagnoses.
    a. Antipsychotics are far more effective with some symptoms of schizophrenia (e.g., positive psychotic symptoms) than others (e.g., negative symptoms).
K. Compliance is a major issue.
  1. True for all pharmacology, but especially psychopharmacology
    a. Impaired insight may go along with some psychiatric disorders.
    b. Impaired ability to stick to a medication schedule may be due to disease-related motivational issues.
    c. Social stigma, including direct pressure from family or peers, may encourage patients to "work it out by themselves" or avoid "mind-altering drugs."

> You will come across some patients' ironic mental schemes that some drugs are "OK" (e.g., marijuana, cocaine, and others), yet "your" medicine is bad because it is "mind-altering". Be prepared!

    d. Positive effects of psychotropic drugs are often delayed.
  2. Quality of your relationship with patient is single strongest predictor of compliance
L. Avoid polypharmacy.
  1. Whenever possible use a single drug class (e.g., one antidepressant for treatment of depression). However, some patients may have treatment-resistant disorders, requiring drug combination strategies, or some subtypes of disorders routinely require two different drug classes (e.g., major depression with psychotic features require an antidepressant and an antipsychotic).

M. Acute treatment ≠ maintenance treatment.
  1. Getting the patient well and keeping the patient well are two different jobs for the medication.
  2. Most major psychiatric disorders tend to *recur* (new episode) or *relapse* (get more symptomatic again before having reached recovery from the initial episode). Once the patient is better acutely, you need to consider the strategy of keeping patient well—whether continued on the same medication, tapering off, or considering different medication for prophylactic treatment.
N. Learn a few drugs from each class well.
  1. The list of psychotropic medications is rather long.
  2. Get to know a few drugs in each treatment class (e.g., antidepressants, antipsychotics, anxiolytics, mood stabilizers) very well. Know their indications, typical doses, typical side effects, and usual problems with drug-drug interactions.
O. Be skeptical of new products and trends (fads?) in prescribing practices.
  1. Avoid being the first (or last) "doctor on your block" to try new medications unless the clinical situation requires it. It may take months or even years to really sort out a new drug's efficacy and toxicity as well as how it compares with previous agents.

 "Never be the first to give the new a try, nor the last to cast the old aside."

P. Remember the heterogeneity of group populations.
  1. Like most medical practice, the empirical base of clinical psychopharmacology rests on studies of patient groups. Individual patients may vary, and a current patient may be an outlier in clinical response, toxicity, or dosage requirements.

 When facing the challenge of heterogeneity in treating patients psychopharmacologically, your viewpoint may be that this is maddening (in the nontechnical sense) or a fun intellectual challenge. The latter perspective is highly recommended!

Q. Clinical indications mentioned through this book may not be the same as United States Food and Drug Administration (FDA)-approved indications. Many drugs are used "off-label" (not the FDA-approved indication). There may be literature or clinical experience to back up the clinical indication, but the pharmaceutical company many not have sponsored studies to prove the drug's effectiveness for that indication to the FDA.

II. Specific Drug Classes

A. Overview
   1. The following is intended as orientation to main types of drugs found in psychiatric settings.
   2. It is neither exhaustive nor a substitute for a good reference text on psychopharmacology.
B. Antipsychotics XX Antipsychotics 1-4
   1. Overview
      a. Comprising first-generation ("typical") antipsychotics and second-generation ("atypical") antipsychotics
      b. First-generation antipsychotics
         i. D_2 receptor antagonists
         ii. Major benefits: lower cost as many generics available
         iii. Major risks: extrapyramidal side effects (EPS) acutely and tardive dyskinesia (TD) with long-term use
         iv. Have been used much less since introduction of second-generation drugs, although recent data question whether the benefit/risk ratio in fact favors a return to first-generation drugs in many cases
      c. Second-generation antipsychotics
         i. D_2 and $5-HT_2$ receptor antagonists
         ii. Major benefits: greatly reduced risk of EPS and TD
         iii. Major risks: metabolic syndrome (see below); elevated triglycerides may be early warning
      d. Indications for all antipsychotics
         i. Psychotic symptoms (as part of many disorders)
         ii. Manic symptoms (as part of bipolar, schizoaffective, or secondary disorders)
         iii. Acute impulse dyscontrol or affective instability or lability (e.g., as part of personality disorders under acute stressors or in dementia or other secondary syndromes, although

safety and efficacy issues are being reviewed in dementia population)

  iv. Acute psychomotor agitation caused by above or other syndromes

  v. Tics, choreiform movements, and some other adventitious movements

  vi. Nausea and vomiting (some agents, such as prochlorperazine [Compazine] are marketed specifically as antiemetics)

  vii. Intractable and disabling hiccoughs

e. Side effects

  i. First- and second-generation drugs may share many side effects as a class but will be annotated as appropriate

  ii. EPS: (more common in first-generations and high-dose risperidone)

    (1) Acute: *dystonia* (sustained muscle contractions that may be painful); *akathisia* (motor restlessness, often manifested as pacing, rocking, or other symmetric/rhythmic motions), and *parkinsonism* (which, like manifestations of idiopathic Parkinson's disease, includes bradykinesia, rigidity, festinating gait, and drooling)

    (2) Delayed (after months or year of exposure: in some cases may not be reversible) *tardive dyskinesia (TD), tardive dystonia,* and *tardive akathisia*

  iii. Neuroleptic malignant syndrome (NMS): rare, potentially life-threatening syndrome, thought to be idiosyncratic drug reaction (see Chapter 7 for more details)

  iv. Anticholinergic effects: dry mouth, constipation, blurry vision, urinary retention, tachycardia, potential to precipitate episode of acute narrow angle glaucoma, delirium

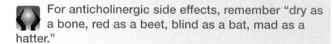 For anticholinergic side effects, remember "dry as a bone, red as a beet, blind as a bat, mad as a hatter."

  v. Orthostatic hypotension (probably related to alpha$_1$-adrenergic blockade)

  vi. Sedation

  vii. Skin: allergic rashes (like many drugs), photosensitivity— such that patients should use ultraviolet skin protectants

    viii. Ocular pigmentation (including pigmentary retinopathy seen with thioridazine above 800 mg/day)

    ix. Galactorrhea (because dopamine inhibits prolactin release from pituitary and antipsychotics block dopamine)

    x. Weight gain (longer-term side effect in some first-generations; clozapine and olanzapine especially among second-generations)

    xi. Nonspecific electrocardiogram (ECG) changes, including ST-segment and T-wave alterations, rarely of clinical significance; prolongation of QT_c, which may be predictive of torsades de pointes arrhythmia risk; in overdose: widening of PR or QT interval or other arrhythmias

    xii. Hepatic toxicity: cholestatic jaundice in low-potency first-generations; all have some risk of elevation of hepatocellular enzymes, usually without clinical significance, except for need to monitor

    xiii. Seizures: lowering seizure threshold is described for nearly all psychotropics (except anticonvulsants)

    xiv. Agranulocytosis: rare, mostly in low-potency phenothiazines among first-generations; clozapine dispensing by pharmacy is contingent on FDA-mandated weekly (or biweekly after 6 months of use) white blood cell (WBC) count and absolute neutrophil count (ANC)

    xv. Sexual dysfunction, including retrograde ejaculation in older low-potency drugs

    xvi. Metabolic syndrome (more common in second-generations)

      (1) Several disorders regarding metabolism at same time, including insulin resistance, obesity—especially truncal (abdominal), elevated blood pressure, elevated triglycerides, and low level of high-density lipoprotein (HDL)

2. First-generation antipsychotics

  a. Pharmacokinetics

    i. All equally effective if given in equivalent doses; potency varies widely

    ii. Relative potency often denoted by comparison with 100-mg chlorpromazine

    iii. Table 16.1 lists examples

    iv. All lipophilic and metabolized hepatically

    v. Half-life varies but in range of at least 18–24 hours (once-daily dosing is usually sufficient and helps compliance)

b. Major area of risk is EPS and TD
3. Second-generation antipsychotics
  a. Pharmacokinetics
    i. Half-life varies extensively from about 7 hours (quetiapine, ziprasidone) to 75 hours (aripiprazole)
    ii. P450 isoenzyme metabolism
  b. Table 16.2 lists examples
  c. With effects beyond dopamine system, putatively somewhat helpful in negative symptoms in schizophrenia; clozapine has been demonstrated to reduce psychotic symptoms in schizophrenic patients resistant to several adequate trials of typical antipsychotics
  d. Availability
    i. Oral (PO)/enteral tube formulations include pills, liquids, or orally disintegrating tablets (depending on specific drug)
    ii. Intramuscular (IM) formulations available for ziprasidone, olanzapine, and aripiprazole; depot formulation available in risperidone only
    iii. Intravenous (IV) use not available (only IV antipsychotic used is haloperidol, a first-generation antipsychotic)
C. Antidepressants XX Antidepressants 1–5
  1. Pharmacokinetics
    a. All lipophilic
    b. Metabolism depends to greater or lesser extent on hepatic oxidation, conjugation, and excretion
    c. Half-life varies but for many they are either long enough or put into extended-release formulations that allow once-a-day dosing in most
  2. Availability
    a. None available in United States in parenteral form, requiring a working gastrointestinal tract and willingness to swallow (or enteral tube), with exception of selegeline skin patch (Emsam)
  3. Mechanism of action
    a. Not fully known, but hypothesized to work in different ways that may drive clinical decisions in more treatment-resistant cases
    b. Extracellular
      i. Presynaptic

TABLE 16.1 Some First-Generation (Typical/Traditional) Antipsychotics XX Antipsychotics 2

Name (Brand Name)	Chemical Class	Approximate Chlorpromazine (CPZ) Equivalents (mg = 100 mg CPZ)	Available Parenterally	Comments
Chlorpromazine (Thorazine)	Aliphatic phenothiazine	100	Yes	IM injections require large amounts of fluid vehicle and may be painful
Mesoridazine (Serentil)	Piperidine phenothiazine	50	Yes	QTc prolongation has limited its usefulness
Thioridazine (Mellaril)	Piperidine phenothiazine	95–100	No	QTc prolongation has limited its usefulness
Fluphenazine (Prolixin)	Piperazine phenothiazine	2	Yes	Available as decanoate
Perphenazine (Trilafon)	Piperazine	8	Yes	
Trifluoperazine (Stelazine)	Piperazine phenothiazine	5	Yes	

Thiothixene (Navane)	Thioxanthene	5	Yes	
Loxapine (Loxitane)	Dibenzoxepine	10–15	Yes	Chemically related to antidepressant amoxapine; some similarities to atypical antipsychotics
Molindone (Moban)	Indolone	10	No	Noted for less risk of weight gain
Droperidol (Inapsine)	Butyrophenone	1–2	Yes	Parenteral only
Haloperidol (Haldol)	Butyrophenone	2–4	Yes	Available as decanoate; sometimes used IV (watch QTc)
Pimozide (Orap)	Diphenylbutylpiperidine	1	No	

| TABLE 16.2 | Second-Generation (Atypical) Antipsychotics: Comparative Properties | | | | | | | XX Antipsychotics 2 |

Name (Brand Name)	Relative potency (mg)	T ½ (hr)	Major Route of Metabolism	Weight Gain	QTc Prolongation	EPS	Prolactin Elevation	Sedation	Metabolic Syndrome Risk
Clozapine (Clozaril)	110	12	CYP 1A2, 2C (minor), 2D6 (minor), 2E1, 3A3/4	+++	+/-	-	+/- to 0	+++	Most
Olanzapine (Zyprexa)	4	30	Glucuronidation CYP 1A2	+++	+/-	+/- to +	+/-	++	Most
Quetiapine (Seroquel)	80	6–7	CYP 3A4	+	+/-	+/- to -	+/-	++	Moderate
Risperidone (Risperdal)	1	20	CYP 2D6 CYP 3A4	+ to ++	+/-	+/- to ++ (dose related)	++	+	Moderate
Ziprasidone (Geodon)	20	7	Aldehyde oxidase	+/-	+ to ++	+/- to +	+/-	+	Low
Aripiprazole (Abilify)	6	75	CYP 2D6 CYP 3A4	+/-	0	+/- to 0	+/-	+	Low

(1) Reuptake inhibition—e.g., tricyclic antidepressants (TCAs), selective serotonin reuptake inhibitors (SSRIs), SNRIs, dopamine-norepinephrine reuptake inhibitors (DNRIs)

(2) Autoreceptor/heteroreceptor inhibition (e.g., mirtazapine)

   ii. Postsynaptic

     (1) $5HT_{1A}$-agonism (e.g., neurotransmitter serotonin)

     (2) $5\text{-}HT_2$ antagonism (e.g., trazodone, nefazodone, mirtazapine)

     (3) Receptor down-regulation (e.g., many antidepressants, electroconvulsive therapy)

  c. Intracellular

    i. Presynaptic

     (1) Mitochondrial monoamine oxidase (MAO) (e.g., MAO inhibitors) (MAOIs)

    ii. Postsynaptic

     (1) Cascade of steps including receptors, G-proteins, c-AMP, protein kinase A, protein kinase C antagonism, cyclic-AMP response element binding (CREB, protein affecting target gene expression), brain-derived neurotropic factor (BDNF)

 d. Agents that are direct agonists (e.g., dopamine agonists such as bromocriptine or amantadine) or that promote release of endogenous catecholamines (e.g., psychostimulants) are less helpful as antidepressants in monotherapy (although some show promise in augmentation strategies)

 e. Table 16.3 lists classes of antidepressants by proposed mechanism of action

4. Indications

 a. Major depressive syndrome as part of major depressive, bipolar, or schizoaffective disorders; secondary mood disorders; dementia; or almost anything else except depressive-like syndrome of hypoactive delirium (may worsen delirium)

 Subtypes of depression (e.g., psychotic depression, melancholia, atypical depression); may have specific implications for choice of antidepressant or need to combine with other agents.

TABLE 16.3

Antidepressant Classes XX Antidepressants 1

Class	Examples
TCA	AMI NTP DMI Imipramine
SNRI	Venlafaxine IR/XR Duloxetine
SSRI	Fluoxetine Sertraline Paroxetine Citalopram Escitalopram Fluvoxamine
5HT-2 antagonists	Trazodone Nefazodone
DNRI	Bupropion IR/SR/XL
MAOI	Tranylcypromine Phenelzine Selegiline skin patch
Noradrenergic and specific serotonergic antidepressant	Mirtazapine

b. Other, less severe depressive syndrome, such as dysthymic disorder, or secondary mood disorders that do not meet criteria for major depressive syndrome (both efficacy and empirical support is lower than for major depression)

c. Panic disorder (best demonstrated: tricyclics, MAOIs, SSRIs)

d. Generalized anxiety disorder (SSRIs, venlafaxine)

e. Social anxiety disorder (MAOIs, SSRIs, venlafaxine)

f. "Positive" symptoms of post-traumatic stress disorder (PTSD) (best demonstrated: tricyclics, MAOIs, SSRIs)

g. Obsessive-compulsive disorder (OCD) (best demonstrated: SSRIs, clomipramine [CMI])

h. Acute cocaine craving (tricyclics, bupropion)

i. Eating disorders, especially bulimia (SSRIs)

j. Attention deficit/hyperactivity disorder (ADHD) (probably; some evidence supports this indication, e.g., bupropion, venlafaxine)

5. Other conditions that may benefit from antidepressants

   a. Prophylaxis of chronic headaches of muscle tension or (some) migraine-spectrum origin (tricyclics, probably SSRIs)

   b. Neuropathic pain syndromes (tricyclics and SNRIs [duloxetine, venlafaxine] more than SSRIs)

   c. Insomnia, primary treatment in transient psychophysiological insomnia, and adjunctive in other insomnias (any sedating antidepressant, e.g., trazodone, amitriptyline [AMI], doxepin, mirtazapine)

   d. Enuresis (most powerfully anticholinergic tricyclics, e.g., AMI, doxepin)

6. Choosing which drug to use

   a. Although most antidepressants may have similar efficacy rates (compared with placebo) in groups with nonpsychotic, nonmelancholic depression (although MAOIs may be more effective than others), individual patients often respond to one agent but not another; hence, the need for medications with different mechanisms of action.

      i. Patient may respond poorly to one class, well to another

      ii. Past response to drug may predict future response

      iii. Family history of response to drug may predict response in patient

      iv. Subtype of depression may influence selection

         (1) Melancholic or inpatients and other severe depressions: tricyclics, MAOIs, ECT, sertraline, venlafaxine, escitalopram

         (2) Seasonal exacerbation: fluoxetine, sertraline, citalopram, mirtazapine, venlafaxine, tranylcypromine, bupropion for acute phase and prevention of recurrence, light therapy

         (3) Atypical features: SSRIs, MAOIs, bupropion

         (4) Psychotic features: antidepressant (best studied are tricyclics and MAOIs) plus antipsychotic, ECT

         (5) Failure of antidepressant monotherapy

            (A) Combination therapy: two antidepressants combined (e.g., SSRI and bupropion)

            (B) Augmentation therapy: drug that itself is not an antidepressant added to an antidepressant to boost its efficacy (e.g., adding lithium, triiodothyronine, buspirone, or psychostimulants)

7. TCAs

a. Side-effect profile

   i. Anticholinergic (tertiary amine more than secondary amine, desipramine [DMI] and nortriptyline [NTP] least offensive)

   ii. Orthostatic hypotension (NTP least offensive)

   iii. Sedation (tertiary amine more than secondary amine)

   iv. Cardiac conduction defects

     (1) TCAs are class 1a antiarrhythmics

     (2) Contraindicated in bifascicular blocks (e.g., left bundle branch block [LBBB] plus first-degree atrioventricular [AV] block)

     (3) Used with caution with worrisome monofascicular blocks (e.g., LBBB or second-degree AV block)

     (4) Increased risk of sudden death (presumably due to ventricular arrhythmias) in patients with coronary artery disease (CAD); hence, use with caution in these patients

     (5) Get ECGs

       (A) Baseline before tricyclics: older patients and those with known heart disease

       (B) During treatment: special attention to PR, QRS, and QT intervals

   v. Potential lethality in overdose: severe cardiac conduction abnormalities, other arrhythmias, seizures, cardiovascular collapse

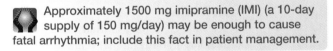 Approximately 1500 mg imipramine (IMI) (a 10-day supply of 150 mg/day) may be enough to cause fatal arrhythmia; include this fact in patient management.

   vi. Sympathomimetic effects: often minimal but prominent in some patients—diaphoresis, postural tremor, anxiety

   vii. Weight gain over longer term

   viii. Sexual dysfunctions, including anorgasmia

   ix. Lowering seizure threshold

b. Active metabolites

   i. DMI is active metabolite of IMI

     (1) Giving IMI results in blood levels of IMI plus DMI

    ii. NTP is active metabolite of AMI

      (1) Giving AMI results in blood levels of AMI plus NTP

  c. Choosing right dosage

    i. Rate of metabolism varies enormously among patients

    ii. Efficacy depends on blood levels

    iii. Data on therapeutic levels in following

      (1) DMI: greater than 125 ng/mL

      (2) NTP: *therapeutic window* 50–150 ng/mL (efficacy best within this range)

      (3) IMI: combined IMI/DMI level of greater than 225 ng/mL

    iv. Other tricyclics: data not reliable

> Do not waste time on drug levels of tricyclics other than DMI, NTP, and IMI, unless you are trying to figure out if patient took overdose or is taking the drug at all.

  d. Choosing which drug to use

    i. DMI and NTP are least sedating and least anticholinergic and have been used most commonly for these reasons

    ii. AMI and doxepin have been commonly used when sedative properties are preferred

    iii. Cost: although generic, DMI and NTP are more expensive than IMI and AMI

  e. Table 16.4 lists examples

8. SNRIs

  a. Examples: venlafaxine, duloxetine

    i. CMI (actually chlorinated imipramine) affects serotonin and norepinephrine. Structurally it is a tricyclic. CMI is sometimes classified as an SNRI; although all TCAs affect serotonin and norepinephrine reuptake, CMI has a more robust effect than the other TCAs. Its more potent effect on serotonin reuptake makes it much more effective in OCD than other TCAs.

  b. Side effects

    i. Similar to those of SSRIs (see below), but can have sustained increase in blood pressure in a small percentage of patients as the dose is raised (thought to be secondary to norepinephrine effect)

  c. May be useful in SSRI failures

Name (Brand Name)	Chemical Class	Typical Dose Range*	Comments

TABLE 16.4 — **Some Tricyclic Antidepressants** — XX Antidepressants 1–2

Name (Brand Name)	Chemical Class	Typical Dose Range*	Comments
NTP (Pamelor, Aventyl)	Secondary amine tricyclic	50–150 mg/day	Therapeutic window of efficacy, in plasma level 50–150 ng/mL
DMI (Norpramin, Pertofrane)	Secondary amine tricyclic	150–300 mg/day	Therapeutic plasma level >125 ng/mL
Protriptyline (Vivactil)	Secondary amine tricyclic	10–40 mg/day	Highly activating (hence its name), which may be a limiting side effect
IMI (Tofranil)	Tertiary amine tricyclic	150–300 mg/day	Therapeutic plasma level >225 ng/mL (combined IMI and DMI level)
AMI (Elavil)	Tertiary amine tricyclic	150–300 mg/day	Therapeutic plasma level unclear, although many laboratories report combined AMI and NTP levels)
Doxepin (Sinequan)	Tertiary amine tricyclic	150–300 mg/day	
CMI (Anafranil)	Tertiary amine tricyclic	150–300 mg/day	Structurally a tricyclic, has tricyclic side effects, is a particularly potent SNRI (used to treat OCD because of the strong serotonin effect compared with other tricyclics)

Some Tricyclic Antidepressants XX Antidepressants 1–2 (continued)			
Name (Brand Name)	Chemical Class	Typical Dose Range*	Comments
Maprotiline (Ludiomil)	Tetracyclic	50–200 mg/day	Most "noradrenergic" of this class of drugs
Amoxapine (Asendin)	Dibenzoxazepine (heterocyclic)	150–300 mg/day	Chemically related to antipsychotic loxapine; may have antipsychotic-like side effects including potential for TD

*Remember enormous variability among patients!

    d. Dose increases more effective in gaining more responders than SSRIs

9. SSRIs

    a. Examples: fluoxetine, sertraline, paroxetine, fluvoxamine, citalopram, escitalopram

    b. Easy to administer based on standard dose ranges; blood levels not needed

    c. Side-effect profile

        i. Anorexia (usually limited), weight loss (those who have anorexia from depression and respond to SSRI will have improved appetite); weight gain can be side effect in longer term

        ii. Insomnia (when patient's depression responds to SSRI, sleep improves); some people feel slightly sedated

        iii. Nausea and (less often) vomiting

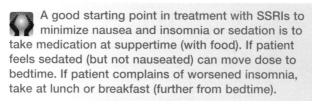

A good starting point in treatment with SSRIs to minimize nausea and insomnia or sedation is to take medication at suppertime (with food). If patient feels sedated (but not nauseated) can move dose to bedtime. If patient complains of worsened insomnia, take at lunch or breakfast (further from bedtime).

iv. Headache
v. Sexual dysfunctions including anorgasmia, ejaculatory delay, decreased libido
vi. Central nervous system (CNS) effects include anxiety, increased arousal or jitteriness, akasthisia or similar states of increased psychomotor activity, delirium (usually in patients with preexisting brain disease)
vii. Inhibition of certain cytochrome P450 isozymes, leading to clinically meaningful (e.g., 100%–400%) rises in blood levels of other drugs metabolized through this system; pay particular attention to risk of interaction with drugs that have narrow therapeutic ranges like *beta blockers* and *warfarin;* SSRIs with less P450 interaction effect are citalopram, escitalopram, venlafaxine, and mirtazepine (see drug-drug interaction section at end of chapter)

 For drug-drug interactions, you may not remember all the interactions, but remember to think about it, and look information up as appropriate.

10. 5-HT$_2$ antagonists
   a. Trazodone (Desyrel)
      i. Long anecdotal experience has led many clinicians to believe less effective than other antidepressants
      ii. Sedating side effect has led to most common use as hypnotic, often administered with stimulating antidepressants like SSRIs or MAOIs
      iii. Other side effects include orthostatic hypotension and (rare but severe) priapism
      iv. Usual hypnotic dosage 25–100 mg qhs, full antidepressant dosage in the 300–600 mg/day range
   b. Nefazodone (only available as generic)
      i. Reports of hepatotoxicity (idiosyncratic reactions with fulminant hepatic necrosis) led to trade-name drug Serzone taken off market
      ii. Generic still available for patients who have done well on it
      iii. Less sedating than trazodone and does not cause orthostatic hypotension in most patients

11. DNRIs

   a. Bupropion (Wellbutrin, Zyban)

      i. Sometimes called a DNRI but actual mechanism of action remains somewhat obscure—although efficacy and tolerability are well established

      ii. Probably as good a choice as SSRI for first-line treatment in uncomplicated outpatient major depression

      iii. Only major antidepressant that probably does *not* treat panic disorder or other primary anxiety disorders

      iv. Seizure risk more significant in immediate release (IR) form than sustained release (SR) or once-a-day extended release (XR) form; target dose 300–450 mg/day

      v. Other potential side effects

         (1) Stimulant-like effects, including psychomotor agitation, insomnia, anxiety, tremor

         (2) Nausea

         (3) Headaches

12. MAOIs

   a. Broad spectrum in neurotransmitter effect; enhancing norepinephrine, serotonin, and dopamine by blocking central MAO

   b. Irreversible inhibitors of monoamine oxidase-A (MAO-A) and monoamine oxidase-B (MAO-B)

      i. Two oral forms marketed: tranycypromine (Parnate) and phenelzine (Nardil) (isocarboxazid [Marplan]) only rarely/intermittently available in United States)

      ii. Hypotension most common side effect, but if food with high amounts of tyramine or sympathomimetic drug consumed, hypertensive crisis may occur

         (1) If MAO-A inhibited in the gut, tyramine is not broken down and causes a release of catecholamines from nerve terminals, resulting in hypertensive crisis

 Clinical presentation of hypertensive crisis is what would be expected from sympathomimetic activity: malignant hypertension (with attendant manifestations including headache, nausea/vomiting, angina, or stroke), tachycardia, diaphoresis, fever, and cardiac arrhythmias.

> Some clinicians give patients a small supply of nifedipine 10 mg, or chlorpromazine 25 mg, to have PRN if symptomatic from dietary indiscretion or other inadvertent ingestion of sympathomimetic amines.

   iii. Other side effects
      (1) Stimulant-like effects, such as insomnia, anxiety, tremor, diaphoresis, myclonic jerks (tranylcypromine more than phenelzine)
      (2) Sexual dysfunctions (impotence, anorgasmia)
      (3) Weight gain
      (4) Anticholinergic effects (although much less than tricyclics)
      (5) Hepatitis (more likely with phenelzine)
  c. Irreversible inhibitors of MAO-B
    i. Oral form selegeline (Eldepryl)
      (1) Used in Parkinson's disease in low doses
      (2) In higher oral doses is antidepressant and blocks MAO-A and MAO-B: same dietary and other precautions as tranylcypromine and phenelzine
    ii. As skin patch selegeline (Emsam) dose of 6 mg/24 hours; avoids MAO-A inhibition in gut and first-pass metabolism; has high bioavailability, thus no dietary restrictions needed; at doses of 9 or 12 mg/24 hours patch, dietary restrictions *are* necessary; pharmacological restrictions as MAO-A and MAO-B inhibitors apply at all skin-patch doses
  d. Reversible inhibitors of monoamine oxidase-A (RIMAs)
    i. Example: moclobemide (Manerix, Aurorix); not available in United States
    ii. Lower propensity to cause hypertensive crisis with high-tyramine foods
13. Norepinephrine and Specific Serotonin Antidepressant
  a. Example: mirtazapine (Remeron)
  b. Side effects: sedation and weight gain most common
    i. As such, not as popular in more medically healthy population
    ii. Very helpful in cachectic, medically ill patients with insomnia; generally in treatment-resistant depression

patients, often as add-on (combination) second antidepressant

c. Mechanism of action

i. Alpha$_2$-autoreceptor presynaptic antagonism: encourages more release of neurotransmitters norepinephrine and serotonin into synaptic cleft, stimulating desired 5-HT$_{1A}$ postsynaptic receptor and adrenergic receptors

ii. 5-HT$_2$ postsynaptic antagonism: antidepressant effect; thus, drug does *not* cause sexual side effect, anxiogenic effects, or insomnia

iii. 5-HT$_3$ postsynaptic antagonism: reduces and treats nausea and diarrhea effect of serotonin in synapse (ondansetron-like activity)

D. Psychostimulants `XX Other Topics 2`

1. Dopaminergic and mixed effects

a. Examples: methylphenidate (Ritalin products of different release/action lengths), dextroamphetamine (Dexedrine), mixed amphetamine salts (Adderall)

i. Actions: facilitate transmission of endogenous catecholamines

ii. Uses

(1) ADHD: improves attention, hyperactivity, cognitive performance

(2) Depressive symptoms: monotherapy not as efficacious as when added to existing antidepressants; helpful in older, medically ill patients without full-fledged major depression, but with prominent anergia, amotivation, and psychomotor slowing

iii. Typical side effects

(1) As predicted for sympathomimetics

(2) Anorexia, other gastrointestinal symptoms, weight loss

(3) Insomnia

2. Norepinephrine reuptake inhibitor

a. Example: atomoxetine (Strattera)

i. Used in ADHD, other uses as above; data in depression disappointing

3. Other

a. Example: modafinil (Provigil)

i. Not typical psychostimulant

ii. Has complex activity fostering catecholamines; also histamine agonist

iii. Classified as a wakefulness promoting agent

iv. Used in narcolepsy, ADHD, and augmentation of antidepressants; for fatigue in medically ill patients

E. Mood stabilizers (thymoleptics) (XX Mood Stabilizers 1-3)

1. Overview

a. Drugs with demonstrated mood-stabilizing efficacy include lithium, carbamazepine (Tegretol/Equetro), and valproic acid (Depakene, Depakote)

b. Other agents have varying amounts of data suggesting they *may be* efficacious but not yet formally classified as mood stabilizers; include calcium channel blockers, oxcarbazepine (Trileptal), zonisamide (Zonegran), atypical antipsychotics, lamotrigine (Lamictal)

c. Some drugs may be more efficacious in one phase of illness compared with another

i. Lamotrigine in bipolar depression more than in mania

ii. Lithium in bipolar mania more than in depression

iii. Typical antipsychotics are antimanic

iv. Atypical antipsychotics may be both antimanic and antidepressive, hence closer to actual "mood-stabilizing" properties

d. Mechanism of action

i. Given wide variety of drug classes, no single principle has been explanatory; e.g., lithium, a cation; lipophilic anticonvulsants acting on any of several neurotransmitter systems

ii. Cation: may compete or substitute at ion channels or receptor sites; lithium potentially affects wide range of neurobiological activity, but most salient effects not known

iii. Anticonvulsant agents in bipolar disorder led to "kindling" theories of mood disorders

(1) Repeated activation (by emotional or biological stressor) of involved neural pathways leads to easier reactivation, or "kindling" — analogous to models of seizure disorders

(2) Unclear whether kindling phenomena are truly relevant to the disease or mechanism or drug actions

    e. Variety of mechanisms may be useful when combining drugs in treatment-resistant cases

2. Indications

    a. Clinical subgrouping may be useful to consider in initial selection of agent in bipolar disorder

       i. Lithium in euphoric mania

      ii. Valproic acid in rapid cycling (four or more mood episodes per year), comorbid substance abuse, dysphoric mania (depressive symptoms in presence of manic symptom, or mixed state)

    b. Use of mood stabilizers in other psychiatric syndromes is mostly anecdotal or some small studies

      i. Long-term treatment of aggressivity (e.g., lithium)

      ii. Reduction of behavioral outbursts in mental retardation (e.g., carbamazepine, valproic acid)

      iii. Reduction of anger attacks or other impulsive/self-destructive behaviors in borderline personality disorder or secondary personality change (e.g., valproic acid)

      iv. Reduction of agitation in dementia (e.g., valproic acid)

      v. Impulse dyscontrol (e.g., anticonvulsants)

    c. Common indications

      i. Bipolar I disorder

        (1) Acute phase: manic or mixed episodes

        (2) Prophylaxis: manic or depressive episodes

        (3) "Coverage" to prevent antidepressant-induced manic swings during treatment of depressive episodes

      ii. Bipolar II disorder and cyclothymia: similar indications but fewer data available

      iii. Unipolar major depression

        (1) Augmentation of antidepressants for acute depression (especially lithium)

        (2) Prophylaxis of recurrent episodes (especially lithium)

      iv. Schizoaffective disorder

        (1) Treatment of mood symptoms analogous to bipolar disorder

        (2) Adjunctive to antipsychotics for psychotic symptoms

      v. Schizophrenia: adjunctive to antipsychotics for psychotic symptoms (e.g., lithium, valproic acid)

d. Time to response

    i. Often 10–14 days after therapeutic amount reached in acute mania

    ii. Hence, common practice to use antipsychotics and other agents initially for more rapid effects

    iii. In more chronic states (e.g., chronic episodic aggressivity) or prophylaxis: evaluate over weeks or months

3. Lithium

    a. A cation, therefore hydrophilic and renally excreted

    b. Administered as salts: lithium carbonate (pill) or lithium citrate (liquid)

    c. Half-life (nearly 24 hours in normal renal function) theoretically allows once-a-day dosing

        i. In practice, peak-level side effects make twice-a-day dosing better tolerated

        ii. Only few patients require dosing three or four times a day to reduce peak side effects (with attendant risk of poor compliance with multiple times of dosing)

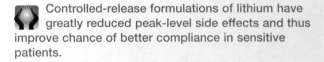 Controlled-release formulations of lithium have greatly reduced peak-level side effects and thus improve chance of better compliance in sensitive patients.

    d. Choosing right dosage

        i. Low therapeutic index: toxicity can occur at levels not very much higher than therapeutic levels.

        ii. Watch conditions or drugs that may raise lithium level.

            (1) Dehydration (e.g., excessive fluid losses on hot day)

            (2) Other hypovolemic states

            (3) Change to low-sodium diet

            (4) Diuretics (especially those such as thiazides that act on distal tubule)

            (5) Nonsteroidal anti-inflammatory drugs (NSAIDs)

            (6) Calcium channel blockers

            (7) Angiotension converting enzyme (ACE) inhibitors

        iii. Published guidelines to therapeutic lithium levels (range 0.6–1.2 mEq/L) are just that; individuals vary enormously in ability to tolerate various levels and level required for efficacy.

iv. Even in same patient, required levels depend on therapeutic goal.

(1) Higher levels (1.0 mEq/L and up) for acute mania

(2) Moderate levels (0.6–0.8 mEq/L) for prophylaxis (although some patients require higher maintenance levels)

(3) Low-moderate levels (0.5 mEq/L or so) for augmentation in unipolar depression

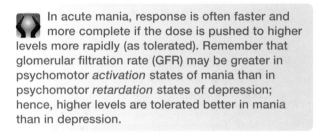 In acute mania, response is often faster and more complete if the dose is pushed to higher levels more rapidly (as tolerated). Remember that glomerular filtration rate (GFR) may be greater in psychomotor *activation* states of mania than in psychomotor *retardation* states of depression; hence, higher levels are tolerated better in mania than in depression.

e. Side effects (common in therapeutic levels moving to toxicities at supratherapeutic levels and overdoses)

i. Gastrointestinal: nausea, diarrhea, anorexia, vomiting

ii. Endocrinological: hypothyroidism, goiter

iii. Cardiac: nonspecific T-wave changes, sinus arrhythmias

iv. Dermatological: exacerbations of acne, psoriasis, or other chronic conditions; rashes of other types (e.g., maculopapular rash, folliculitis, exfoliative dermatitis)

v. Renal: nephrogenic diabetes insipidus, proteinuria (which can rarely reach nephrotic syndrome levels), elevated serum creatinine/renal failure (rare except at toxic lithium levels)

vi. Hematological: benign leukocyctosis

vii. Neurological: tremor (typically position-holding), cognitive or psychomotor slowing, and neuromuscular irritability, dysarthria, ataxia, delirium, seizures (these latter symptoms all being signs of worrisome toxicity)

viii. Over longer time: watch thyroid and renal dysfunction

 When lithium overall helpful, but need to manage side effects, consider options:

(1) *Peak side effects:* decrease dose or divide doses
(2) *Nephrogenic diabetes insipidus:* thiazides or amiloride (but decrease dose to maintain same lithium level)
(3) *Tremor:* beta-adrenergic blockers
(4) *Hypothyroidism:* thyroid replacement hormone
  f. Suggestions on health monitoring in addition to obtaining appropriate lithium levels (in young and otherwise healthy):
  i. Screening, then annual or biannual urinalysis
  ii. Serum creatinine levels
  iii. Thyroid-stimulating hormone (TSH) levels
4. Carbamazepine
  a. Indications
  i. May be effective in patients for whom lithium is ineffective or intolerable—often with fewer CNS side effects at commonly used blood levels
  b. Choosing right dosage
  i. Therapeutic range of levels was established for epilepsy.
  ii. These are rough guides only for psychiatric use. Some patients show benefit at low levels (especially in combination with lithium and other drugs); others tolerate and get additional benefit from high levels.

In use of carbamazepine for psychiatric purposes, it appears that pushing dose up to beginning of side effects is a clinically useful way of determining optimal doses. Levels, as with most anticonvulsants except valproate, are established for seizure control, not for psychiatric uses.

  iii. Carbamazepine induces its own (and certain other drug) metabolism, and levels may drop about 2 weeks out—requiring a modest increase of dose.
  c. Side effects
  i. Neurological: sedation, ataxia, dysarthria, delirium
  ii. Hematological: benign dyscrasias (particularly leukopenia), which should not be confused with feared, but rarely occurring, idiosyncratic severe cell line depletions including aplastic anemia
  iii. Gastrointestinal: nausea, dyspepsia

iv. Cardiac: conduction system disturbances (carbamazepine is structurally related to tricyclic antidepressants)
v. Dermatological: rashes, from benign to exfoliative syndromes
vi. Hepatic: hepatitis
5. Valproic acid
   a. Indications
      i. Similar psychiatric indications as carbamazepine and more data available
      ii. Divalproex and valproate sodium in body form valproic acid
      iii. Forms
         (1) Depakote (divalproex sodium)
         (2) Depakene (valproic acid)
         (3) Depacon (IV valporate sodium)
   b. Choosing right dosage
      i. Loading strategies may allow more rapid dosing in acute states (e.g., 20 mg/kg/day)
      ii. Levels are more reliable for therapeutic effect than carbamazepine; usual range of valproic acid level is 50–100 mcg/mL, up to 125 mcg/mL in mania
   c. Side effects
      i. Neurological: tremor, somnolence initially
      ii. Hematological: thrombocytopenia
      iii. Metabolic: weight gain, edema
      iv. Gastrointestinal: nausea (less with divalproex form)
      v. Skin: hair loss (possibly less with ER form)
      vi. Hepatic: hepatitis—mostly in children
6. Lamotrigine (Lamictal)
   a. Indications
      i. Mania maintenance (after manic episode, preventing recurrence of mania; although less effective in preventing mania than preventing depressive episodes)
      ii. Depression maintenance (after depressive episode, preventing recurrence of depression)
      iii. Bipolar depression (appears effective)
   b. Side effects
      i. Dermatological: serious rash (Stevens-Johnson syndrome, toxic epidermal necrolysis)

  (1) Epilepsy trials (adjunctive to other drugs)
    (A) Children (<16 years) 8/1000
    (B) Adults 3/1000
  (2) Bipolar trials (adults)
    (A) Monotherapy 0.3/1000
    (B) Adjunctive therapy 1.3/1000
  (3) Increased risk of serious rash
    (A) Co-administration with valproate
    (B) Exceeding recommended initial dose
    (C) Exceeding recommended dose escalation
  ii. Neurological: dizziness, ataxia
  iii. Gastrointestinal: nausea
c. Dosing
  i. Slow titration in bipolar trials has reduced risk of rash originally present in epilepsy trials
  ii. Follow recommended dosing suggested for monotherapy, coprescription with metabolic inhibiting drugs, and coprescription with metabolic inducing drugs
F. Anxiolytics (XX Anxiolytics 1–5)
  1. Benzodiazepines
    a. Overview
      i. Most popular of all anxiolytics: efficacy and relatively benign side-effect profile
        (1) Remember that other agents such as antidepressants should be the mainstay of longer-term treatment for most patients
      ii. Relative safety in overdose
    b. Mechanism of action
      i. Agonists at sites in benzodiazepine–gamma-aminobutyric acid (GABA) receptor complex, augmenting activity of inhibitory neurotransmitter GABA
    c. Indications
      i. Primary treatment for anxiety symptoms in panic disorder, generalized anxiety disorder, situation-specific anxiety (e.g., associated with acute medical illnesses, procedures, hospitalizations)
      ii. Adjunctive treatment for anxiety symptoms in wide range of other conditions, most notably major depression

iii. Insomnia: either as primary treatment (e.g., transient psychophysiological insomnia) or as adjunct during initial treatment of mood, psychotic, and other disorders

iv. Adjunctive treatment of psychomotor agitation in acute psychotic or manic states (benzodiazepine use may allow effective acute management with less overall antipsychotic exposure)

v. Antipsychotic-induced akathisia, although other agents (e.g., beta blockers) are usually preferable

vi. Primary treatment of alcohol, barbiturate, or benzodiazepine withdrawal (cross-tolerance among benzodiazepines, barbiturates, and alcohol leads to lessened withdrawal symptoms when administering any of these)

vii. Other uses that exploit properties
   (1) Muscle relaxation (e.g., diazepam for muscle spasms after acute back injury)
   (2) Sedative/hypnotic/amnestic effects (e.g., midazolam for brief medical procedures)

d. Side effects

i. Neurological: sedation, dysarthria, ataxia (beware of increased risk of falls, especially in the elderly) delirium, hallucinosis

ii. Psychiatric: cognitive slowing, amnesia, or global impairment (i.e., delirium); disinhibition (increased impulsivity or aggressivity, akin to what might be seen in ethanol intoxication)

iii. Dependency: patients taking sufficient doses for long enough will develop physiological dependency; withdrawal symptoms resembling those of alcohol or barbiturate withdrawal; patients may also become psychologically dependent on benzodiazepines; they become accustomed to (or enjoy) feelings drug induces—may seek higher doses or resist attempts to decrease or stop drug intake

iv. Remarkably few other side effects; effects on pulse, blood pressure, cardiac output, and respiratory function are minimal in most situations except severe overdoses and rapid IV administrations

e. Choosing which drug to use
i. Numerous choices (Table 16.5)

TABLE 16.5	Estimated Dosage Equivalents for Selected Benzodiazepines	
Generic Name (Brand Name)		**Dosage (mg)**
Alprazolam (Xanax)		1.0
Chlordiazepoxide (Librium)		50
Clonazepam (Klonopin)		0.5
Clorazepate (Tranxene)		15
Diazepam (Valium)		10
Flurazepam (Dalmane)		30
Lorazepam (Ativan)		2
Oxazepam (Serax)		30
Temazepam (Restoril)		20
Triazolam (Halcion)		0.25

ii. All probably equally effective at equivalent doses
iii. All have common therapeutic properties as anxiolytics, hypnotics, and muscle relaxants
iv. Vary in pharmacokinetics, including half-life and presence of active metabolites (which may prolong effective half-life even more)

Lorazepam is a high-potency benzodiazepine. Because of its useful absorption and metabolism characteristics, make lorazepam one of the benzodiazepines you become experienced with and comfortable prescribing. Lorazepam is:

(1) Available in oral and parenteral forms.
(2) The only benzodiazepine that is consistently well absorbed intramuscularly (excellent in emergent situations).
(3) One of the few that is metabolized by direct conjugation, not requiring hepatic oxidation, and does not have active metabolites.

2. Buspirone (BuSpar)
   a. Unique anxiolytic
      i. Not sedating

     ii. Does not cause physiological dependency

     iii. Does not have acute effects on anxiety like a benzodiazepine

  b. May be useful augmentation to antidepressant (due to 5-HT$_{1A}$ partial agonism)

  c. Has been used for anxiety, depressive, and secondary mental disorders

3. Sedating antihistamines

  a. Examples: diphenhydramine, hydroxyzine, promethazine

  b. Sometimes used in patients with substance abuse histories for anxiety (due to less risk of physiological dependency)

  c. Not as effective for anxiety as other agents mentioned

G. Benzodiazepine antagonist

  1. Example: flumazenil

H. Alpha antagonist

  1. Example: prazosin (Minipress)

    a. Used in treatment of nightmares in post-traumatic stress disorder

I. Alpha$_2$-adrenergic agonist

  1. Examples: clonidine (Catapres), guanfacine (Tenex)

  2. Used in treatment of nightmares in post-traumatic stress disorder

  3. Clonidine also used in treatment of ADHD with stimulants and symptom control in opioid withdrawal

J. Non-benzodiazepine sedative hypnotics

  1. Examples: zolpidem (Ambien), eszopiclone (Lunesta), zaleplon (Sonata)

  2. Appear to involve benzodiazepine-GABA receptor complex

  3. Not necessarily free of benzodiazepine risks and side effects

> Zaleplon may not work as well if patient has been previously exposed to zolpidem.

K. Antiparkinson drugs

  1. Anticholinergics XX Anticholinergics 1

    a. Benztropine (Cogentin)

      i. Has advantage of IM form and oral form

    b. Trihexyphenidyl (Artane)

    c. Diphenhydramine (Benadryl)

      i. Has advantage of IM and IV use

  2. Dopamine agonists

    a. Amantadine (Symmetrel)

        i. May be especially useful when needing to avoid anticholinergic side effects in treating EPS; useful in akasthisia; sometimes antidepressant augmentation

    b. Pergolide (Permax), pramipexole (Mirapex), ropinirole (Requip)

        i. Have been used in augmentation of antidepressants and in Parkinson's disease and restless leg syndrome

L. Opioid-dependence drugs

  1. Methadone

    a. Opioid with excellent bioavailability in oral dosing and long half-life that makes it useful in:

        i. Offering continuous pain relief.

        ii. Slow dosage reduction to withdraw patients from opioids.

        iii. Chronic administration in comprehensive outpatient drug dependence treatment ("methadone maintenance programs").

    b. Has clearly demonstrated effectiveness in reducing relapse and improving function in patients with opioid dependence

  2. Buprenorphine: partial opioid agonist and antagonist actions

    a. Suboxone: buprenorphine and naloxone (used in less supervised settings: if used intravenously, would cause opioid withdrawal)

    b. Subutex: buprenorphine alone

M. Opioid antagonist

  1. Naloxone (Narcan) [see naltrexone (Revia) under alcohol dependence drug]

    a. If given intravenously, causes rapid but brief opioid withdrawal: useful in opioid intoxication (e.g., following overdose)

N. Alcohol-dependence drugs

  1. Disulfiram (Antabuse) causes *aversive reaction* to alcohol if consumed.

    a. Metabolism of alcohol

        i. Alcohol – (1) → acetaldehyde – (2) → acetic acid

        ii. Enzyme (1) is alcohol dehydrogenase

        iii. Enzyme (2) is acetaldehyde dehydrogenase

    b. Disulfiram inhibits acetaldehyde dehydrogenase, causing high levels of acetaldehyde if alcohol is consumed → flushing, nausea, vomiting, increased heart rate, shortness of breath

2. Naltrexone: *reduces "reward"* of alcohol consumption (and other behaviors) by blocking opioid receptors (which are stimulated by alcohol consumption)
   a. Revia: oral form
   b. Vivitrol: long-acting depot IM form
3. Acamprosate (Campral): may *reduce "craving"* that occurs from increased glutamate (excitatory amino acid) during abstinence
   a. Thought to work by re-establishing balance between *excitatory* glutamate and *inhibitory* GABA that is thought to be disrupted in alcoholism

O. Dementia drugs
   1. Cholinesterase inhibitors
      a. Differentiated in terms of selectivity of acetylcholinesterase (A) versus butyrylcholinesterase (B) inhibition—both found in CNS, but latter also found in liver and plasma
         i. Tacrine (Cognex): B > A
         ii. Donepezil (Aricept): B > A
         iii. Rivastigmine (Exelon): A > B
         iv. Galantamine (Razadyne): A > B
      b. Despite tacrine and donepezil being similar in effect on cholinesterase enzymes, donepezil is very well tolerated and has few drug-drug interactions, whereas tacrine is notable for risk of liver toxicity.
      c. Enhance cholinergic function found to be deficient in dementia
      d. May slow decline of patient
   2. N-methyl-D-aspartate (NMDA) antagonist
      a. Antagonist to NMDA receptor
         i. Stimulation of NMDA receptor by glutamate thought to contribute to symptoms of Alzheimer's disease, by excessive Ca++ influx, causing neuronal death.
      b. Memantine (Namenda)
         i. Useful in moderate to severe Alzheimer's disease
         ii. Added to donepezil, may have additive benefits

P. Beta-adrenergic blockers XX Other Topics
   1. Examples: propranolol (Inderal), nadolol (Corgard), pindolol (Visken), atenolol (Tenormin)
   2. Major psychiatric uses
      a. Neuroleptic-induced akathisia
      b. Peripheral manifestations of situational anxiety or panic

    c. Reduction of violence in brain-injured patients

    d. Pindolol has presynaptic 5-HT$_{1A}$ antagonism that promotes more release of serotonin into the synaptic cleft when used with an SSRI, hastening antidepressant response

Q. Thyroid hormones

  1. Major psychiatric uses beyond obvious treatment of hypothyroidism and lithium-induced goiter (even without hypothyroidism) are:

    a. Treatment of subclinical hypothyroidism (which may overlap in symptoms with depression).

    b. Augmentation of antidepressants or ECT.

    c. Reduction of rapid cycling in bipolar disorder.

  2. Predominance of literature differentiates these two as follows:

    a. T$_3$ (Cytomel, T$_{1/2}$ ≈ 2 days): more useful for augmentation of antidepressants or ECT—probably also has direct pharmacological effect beyond hormone replacement

    b. T$_4$ (Synthroid, T$_{1/2}$ ≈ 6–7 days): more useful for subclinical hypothyroidism and in treatment of rapid cycling (which may have higher incidence of elevated TSH than non-rapid cycling)

III. Cytochrome P-450 Drug-Drug Interactions

  A. A complete listing of known P-450 interactions is beyond the scope of this book.

  B. Some of the interactions are covered in Tables 16.6 through 16.8.

  C. Especially look at the varying degree of isoenzyme inhibition caused by commonly used antidepressant in Table 16.6.

  D. Match common substrates presented in Table 16.7 to antidepressant selected in Table 16.6.

 MENTOR TIPS DIGEST

- You will come across some patients' ironic mental schemes that some drugs are "OK" (e.g., marijuana, cocaine, and others), yet "your" medicine is bad because it is "mind-altering". Be prepared!
- "Never be the first to give the new a try, nor the last to cast the old aside."

TABLE 16.6 Common Antidepressants and Cytochrome P-450 Isoenzyme Inhibition (XX Antidepressants ↑)					
Name (Brand Name)	3A4	2D6	2C19	2C9	1A2
Duloxetine (Cymbalta)	0	XX	0?	0	0/X
Escitalopram (Lexapro)	0	0/X	0	0	0
Citalopram (Celexa)	0	X	0	0	X
Fluoxetine (Prozac)	XX	XXX	XX	XX	X
Paroxetine (Paxil)	X	XXX	X	X	X
Sertraline (Zoloft)	X	X	XX	X	X
Bupropion (Welbutrin, Zyban)	0	XXX	0	0	0
Venlafaxine (Effexor)	0	X	0	0	0
Mirtazapine (Remeron)	X	X	0	0	0
Nefazodone	XXX	0	0	0	0
Fluvoxamine (Luvox)	XXX	0	XXX	0	XXX

Key: X = Low
XX = Moderate
XXX = Strong

• When facing the challenge of heterogeneity in treating patients psycho-pharmacologically, your viewpoint may be that this is maddening (in the nontechnical sense) or a fun intellectual challenge. The latter perspective is highly recommended!
• For anticholinergic side effects remember "dry as a bone, red as a beet, blind as a bat, mad as a hatter"
• Subtypes of depression (e.g., psychotic depression, melancholia, atypical depression), may have specific implications for choice of antidepressant or need to combine with other agents.
• Approximately 1500 mg IMI (a 10-day supply of 150 mg/day) may be enough to cause fatal arrhythmia; include this fact in patient management.
• Do not waste time on drug levels of tricyclics other than DMI, NTP, and IMI, unless you are trying to figure out if patient took overdose or is taking the drug at all.

TABLE 16.7 — Common Substrate Cytochrome P-450 Metabolic Pathways

3A4	3A4	2D6	2C19	2C9	1A2
Dextromethorphan	Diltiazem	Codeine	Lansoprazole	Diclofenac	AMI
Erythromycin	Nifedipine	Dextromethorphan	Omeprazole	Ibuprofen	IMI
Haloperidol	Verapamil	DMI	Pantoprazole	Naproxen	CMI
Imipramine	Indinavir	NTP	Rabeprazole	Piroxicam	Clozapine
Methadone	Nelfinavir	Fluoxetine	Citalopram	Tolbutamide	Caffeine
Prednisone	Ritonavir	Paroxetine	Diazepam	AMI	Cyclobenzaprine
Sertraline	Saquinavir	Fluvoxamine	Imipramine	Celecoxib	Estradiol
Tamoxifen	Carbamazepine	Venlafaxine	Mephenytoin	Fluoxetine	Haloperidol
Alprazolam	Cisapride	Propranolol	R-warfarin	Phenytoin	Acetaminophen
Diazepam	Citalopram	Metoprolol		Sulfamethoxazole	Propranolol
Midazolam	CMI	Timolol		Tamoxifen	Theophylline
Triazolam	Clonazepam	Perphenazine		S-warfarin	Duloxetine
	Cyclobenzaprine	Risperidone			
	cyclosporine	Thioridazine			
		Tamoxifen			
		Tramadol			
		Duloxetine			

TABLE 16.8	Common Inducers and Inhibitors of Cytochrome P-450 (CYP) Isoenzymes	
Isoenzyme	**Inducers**	**Inhibitors**
CYP 3A3/4	Rifampin Rifabutin Dexamethasone Phenytoin Carbamazepine Barbiturates Ritonavir St John's wort	Fluvoxamine Fluoxetine Haloperidol Omeprazole Sertraline Ketoconazole Itraconazole Macrolide antibiotics (not Azithromycin) Nefazodone Amiodarone Cimetidine Grapefruit juice (naringin) HIV protease inhibitors
CYP 2D6	Phenytoin	Quinine Quinidine Paroxetine Fluoxetine Chlorpromazine Fluphenazine Haloperidol Perphenazine Mesoridazine Sertraline
CYP 2C19	Norethindrone Carbamazepine Rifampin	Ticlopidine Paroxetine Omeprazole Lansoprazole Ketoconazole Fluvoxamine Fluoxetine Felbamate Cimetidine

(continued on page 268)

TABLE 16.8	Common Inducers and Inhibitors of Cytochrome P-450 (CYP) Isoenzymes (continued)	
Isoenzyme	**Inducers**	**Inhibitors**
CYP 2C9	Rifampin Phenobarbital	Amiodarone Fluconazole Fluoxetine Fluvastatin Isoniazid Metronidazole Paroxetine Zafirlukast
CYP 1A2	Carbamazepine Cigarette smoking Cruciferous vegetables Cannabis Barbiturates Char-grilled meat Rifampin	Ciprofloxacin Fluvoxamine Paroxetine Cimetidine Ofloxacin Ticlopidine
CYP 2E1	Ethanol (chronic) Isoniazid	Disulfiram Thioridazine

- A good starting point in treatment with SSRIs to minimize nausea and insomnia or sedation is to take medication at suppertime (with food). If patient feels sedated leave there. If patient complains of worsened insomnia, take at lunch or breakfast (further from bedtime).
- For drug-drug interactions, you may not remember all the interactions, but remember to think about it, and look information up as appropriate.
- Clinical presentation of hypertensive crisis is what would be expected from sympathomimetic activity: malignant hypertension (with attendant manifestations including headache, nausea/vomiting, angina, or stroke), tachycardia, diaphoresis, fever, and cardiac arrhythmias.

- Some clinicians give patients a small supply of nifedipine 10 mg, or chlorpromazine 25 mg, to have PRN if symptomatic from dietary indiscretion, or inadvertent. sympathomimetic amines.
- Controlled-release formulations of lithium have greatly reduced peak-level side effects and thus improve chance of better compliance in sensitive patients.
- In acute mania, response is often faster and more complete if dose is pushed to higher levels more rapidly (as tolerated). Remember that glomerular filtration rate (GFR) may be greater in psychomotor *activation* states of mania than in psychomotor *retardation* states of depression; hence higher levels are tolerated better in mania than in depression.
- When lithium overall helpful, but need to manage side effects, consider options (as discussed in text).
- In use of carbamazepine for psychiatric purposes, it appears that pushing dose up to beginning of side effects is a clinically useful way of determining optimal doses. Levels, as with most anticonvulsants (except valproate), are established for seizure control, not for psychiatric uses.
- Lorazepam is a high-potency benzodiazepine. Because of its useful absorption and metabolism characteristics, make lorazepam one of the benzodiazepines you become experienced with and comfortable prescribing.
- Zaleplon may not work as well if patient has been previously exposed to zolpidem.

Resources

Guttmacher LB. Concise guide to psychopharmacology and electroconvulsive therapy. Washington D.C., American Psychiatric Press Inc., 1994, pp. 1–8.

Indiana University Department of Medicine, Division of Clinical Pharmacology, Drug Interactions Web site.
http://www.medicine.iupui.edu/flockhart/
Excellent drug-drug interactions Web site.

Pies RW. Handbook of essential psychopharmacology, 2nd ed. Washington D.C., American Psychiatric Press, 2005.

Stahl SM. Essential psychopharmacology, 2nd ed. Cambridge University Press, Cambridge, United Kingdom, 2000.

Chapter Self-Test Questions

Circle the correct answer. After you have responded to the questions, check your answers in Appendix A.

1. In severe major depression with melancholia, which of the following is likely to be more effective in treating depression?

   a. Lithium

   b. Lorazepam

   c. Paroxetine

   d. Venlafaxine

2. Which of the following best represents the concept that if a close relative of the patient has had an excellent response to a drug, your patient may have an excellent response to the same drug?

   a. Pharmacodynamics

   b. Pharmacogenetics

   c. Pharmacokinetics

   d. Pharmacotherapy

3. Compliance is a major issue in all pharmacology. Which of the following reasons best exemplifies problems with compliance that are especially true of patients with a psychiatric diagnosis?

   a. Cost factors in obtaining medication

   b. Impaired ability to stick to a medication schedule due to disease-related motivational issues

   c. Multiple doses per day

   d. Problems remembering to take medication

4. Which of the following is the term for a new episode of a disorder that has been experienced in the past?

a. Recovery

b. Recurrence

c. Relapse

d. Remission

5. The term for becoming more symptomatic again before having reached recovery stage of an episode is:

a. Recurrence.

b. Relapse.

c. Remission.

d. Response.

 See the testbank CD for more self-test questions.

OTHER SOMATIC THERAPIES

Michael R. Privitera, MD, MS, and Jeffrey M. Lyness, MD

I. Overview

  A. Somatic therapies refer to the "biological" treatments in psychiatry, as contrasted to psychotherapy and other psychosocial treatments.

  B. Within somatic therapy category is pharmacotherapy.

  C. Hence, this chapter refers to biological treatments other than pharmacological in the treatment of psychiatric disorders.

II. Electroconvulsive Therapy (ECT) XX ECT 1-4

  A. Seizure itself is what has therapeutic value, not method of induction

   1. Although broadly categorized as "neuromodulation" treatments in psychiatry (see below), emphasis on seizure itself as therapeutic suggests listing ECT in its own category

  B. Early history, use of various methods of seizure induction

   1. One example: "insulin shock"—used insulin-induced hypoglycemia to induce a seizure; abandoned decades ago due to obvious risks

  C. 1938: Cerletti and Bini used electrical stimulation applied to the scalp to induce seizure; much more reliable and safe than other methods

  D. Efficacy of ECT, absence of other effective treatments, and reimbursibility of procedure led to overuse; overuse and lack of anesthesia (increased risk of fractures during seizure, lack of sedation) led to some deserved bad press in early days, as the procedure was fairly barbaric.

  E. Institution of anesthesia, sedation, and refinement of techniques have made ECT a very safe and effective treatment—no longer deserving of bad press

F. ECT is procedure; requires a consent; pros and cons should be discussed openly among patient, clinicians, and family members
G. Mechanism of action
   1. Not exactly known (no more exactly than how any antidepressant works)
   2. Electrical stimulation is safest and most reproducible way to induce seizure
   3. Seizures → outpouring of catecholamines and many other (most other?) neurotransmitters
   4. Course of ECT → down-regulation of beta-adrenergic receptors (similar to what happens with antidepressants)
H. Indications
   1. Efficacy clearly demonstrated for unipolar and bipolar depression
      a. Particularly melancholic and psychotic subtypes
   2. Often reserved for those intolerant or unresponsive to medications
   3. May be treatment of first choice in psychotic depression and where most rapid and reliable antidepressant response is essential (e.g., intractably suicidal patient; patient requiring nasogastric/intravenous [IV] nutrition/fluids due to cessation of oral intake)
   4. Other uses
      a. Intractable mania
      b. Intractable psychotic symptoms in schizophrenia or schizoaffective disorder (often requires greater number of treatments [~12–20])
      c. Catatonic syndromes
      d. Parkinson's disease (although rapid relapse rates)
   5. Administration
      a. Acute course is usually 6–12 treatments (but may vary depending on tolerability and treatment response)
      b. Inpatient or outpatient basis
      c. In United States usually three times per week
      d. ECT treatment room usually staffed with psychiatrist, anesthesiologist, and psychiatric nurse
      e. Patient anesthetized with IV short-acting agent, usually barbiturate-like thiopental or methohexital, although propofol is gaining proponents

f. Patient "bagged" (ventilated) with oxygen through a face mask (intubation needed only for patients requiring special ventilatory support due to pulmonary disease, airway obstruction, or other special circumstance)

g. Succinylcholine given IV, then patient observed for maximum muscle paralysis of depolarization-induced muscle fasciculations (may be assessed by use of cutaneous nerve stimulator)

h. Electroencephalogram (EEG) leads placed to record electrical activity to document seizure and length

i. ECT stimulus given via scalp placement chosen by psychiatrist; e.g., bitemporal, unilateral, or bifrontal positions

j. Blood pressure cuff inflated above systolic blood pressure on one arm (before succinylcholine given) to be able to witness (confirm) "unmodified" motor movement of that extremity by seizure

k. Seizure duration intended to be at least 25–30 seconds to be adequately therapeutic; 45–90 seconds is typical range

l. Whole procedure takes about 5 minutes; patient wakens rapidly and is monitored in recovery area until full consciousness regained

m. ECT excellent treatment for *acute phase* of major depression (response rates 80%–90%) but episodes recur unless prevention instituted

  i. Either *maintenance ECT* [spread frequency of treatments slowly out to once per month] indefinitely, or

  ii. *Medication prophylaxis* [best evidence is combination of nortriptyline plus lithium]

6. Side effects

a. Anesthetized, patients feel no pain and do not remember treatment from point anesthetic given

b. Some amount of grogginess not uncommon for several hours after treatment (although many do not experience this)

c. Some sensitive patients can become delirious after treatment; if occurs, usually does so later in treatment course as this and other cognitive side effects are often cumulative with the series of treatments

d. Anesthesia side-effects risk (although seizure may contribute)

    i. Nausea and headache
    ii. Risk of death (~1/10,000 ECT treatments), which is actually less than the risk of brief general anesthesia procedures for other indications and less than the risk of death in context of inadequately treated severe depression

e. Memory
    i. Some retrograde amnesia, mostly anterograde amnesia
    ii. Usually clears within several weeks after last ECT treatment

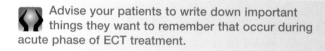

> Advise your patients to write down important things they want to remember that occur during acute phase of ECT treatment.

    iii. More common in acute series than in maintenance treatments (as treatments are further apart with less accumulation of cognitive impact)

> Memory impairments due to major depression *improve with ECT*; make sure to explain this anticipated benefit to your patient.

f. Numerous studies: *no* permanent cognitive or neuropsychological impairments (despite claims of a number of publicly visible anti-ECT figures)

g. Neuroimaging studies: no anatomic changes or lesions even in patients with >100 treatments over lifetime

h. Cognitive deficits
    i. Neither associated with nor required for treatment response
    ii. Deficits with bilateral ECT are greater than for unilateral ECT
    iii. Greater with electric current above seizure threshold

i. Efficacy
    i. Efficacy of bilateral ECT (one stimulus electrode over each hemisphere) greater than that of unilateral ECT (both stimulus electrodes over nondominant hemisphere)
    ii. Higher-dose (higher current) unilateral ECT more efficacious than lower-dose unilateral ECT

iii. Higher-dose bilateral ECT ≈ lower-dose bilateral ECT in efficacy, both greater than in any unilateral treatment course

> Although low-dose bilateral ECT has slightly better efficacy than high-dose unilateral ECT, efficacy is close enough that clinically high-dose unilateral ECT is a good option for many patients sensitive to cognitive side effects of bilateral ECT.

III. Psychosurgery
  A. Ablative
    1. Overview
      a. Using neurosurgical techniques that make permanent changes surgically
      b. Long history, with much bad press in some cases that remains to this day, deservedly so given abuses decades ago
      c. Modern techniques and more restrictive application have led to gradual reappraisal of the role of psychosurgery for selected severely ill patients
    2. Prefrontal lobotomy (severing prefrontal region from rest of brain (1935, Moniz and Lima; Moniz received Nobel Prize for this in 1949)
      a. Used in severe depression and obsessive-compulsive disorder (OCD)
      b. Evolved from crude to stereotactic procedure
    3. "Ice pick lobotomy" (Freeman, late 1930s to 1950s)
      a. Ice pick and rubber mallet (instead of surgical technique of lobotomy), brief/minimal anesthesia (sometimes ECT for anesthesia)
      b. Left virtually no scars, heralded as great advance as if minimally invasive (was anything but minimally invasive)
      c. Reduced spontaneity, calmed, change in personality, reduced sexual drive
      d. Used indiscriminately for large numbers of patients, led to deserved bad press and eventual abandonment of the procedure
    4. Tractotomy
      a. Stereotactic subcaudate tractotomy
      b. Used in treatment-resistant depression, bipolar affective disorder

5. Cingulotomy (1995, Baer)
   a. Lesion in cingulum, near corpus callosum
   b. OCD treatment of last resort
   c. Usually goes before an ethics board for review before procedure
B. Neuromodulation
   1. Overview
      a. Using currents to change electrical environment of various targeted nerves or brain tissue to get desired effect, hence reversible
   2. Vagus nerve stimulation (VNS)
      a. Adapted in psychiatry from work in treatment of refractory epilepsy, with mood improvement
      b. FDA approved for treatment of depression (although controversy over data sufficient that many insurance companies are not currently paying for this procedure)
      c. Appears that acute effects not as robust as longer-term improvements
      d. Vagus nerve is mixed motor and sensory nerve
         i. Left vagus: 80% afferent sensory; afferents project to nucleus tractus solitarius (NTS) in the brainstem, which in turn projects to midline raphe nuclei and locus coeruleus (wherein antiseizure and neuropsychiatric effects occur)
      e. Metal coil wrapped around left vagus nerve in cervical region
      f. Pulse generator implanted in left chest wall to deliver stimulation
   3. Deep brain stimulation
      a. Adapted from work in neurology for Parkinson's disease, essential tremor, and dystonia
      b. Still experimental; small studies suggest significant improvement in treatment-resistant depression and OCD
      c. Brodmann area 25 (subgenual cingulate region) found to be hyperactive in many patients with major depression, as foundation for target of stimulation in depressed patients
      d. Thin electrode placed stereotactically to stimulate area 25, reducing overactivity
      e. Pulse generator implanted in chest wall

IV. Nonsurgical Neuromodulation

A. Repetitive transcranial magnetic stimulation (rTMS)
  1. Still experimental
  2. Noninvasive; anesthesia not needed
  3. Causes electrical activity in nerve cells by applying alternating magnetic fields to skull
  4. Technology allowing multiple trains of stimulation per second relates to term "repetitive"
  5. Subseizure stimulus works better in nonpsychotic depression than in psychotic depression
  6. Above seizure stimulus rTMS (i.e., use of magnetic currents strong enough to induce seizure) being examined as alternative to ECT; however, information currently still unclear as anesthesia needed for same purposes used in ECT
  7. Focus of stimulus based on purported abnormalities in illness states
    a. Depression: underactive left prefrontal cortex
    b. Anxiety states: overactive right prefrontal cortex
    c. OCD: overactive cingulate gyrus
B. Transcranial electrical stimulation
  1. Target is hypothalamus, brainstem
  2. May work by increasing serotonin, reduced acetylcholine and norepinephrine
  3. Limited evidence that this procedure may have some calming and mood-stabilizing properties

V. Light Therapy

A. Brightness and quality of ambient light influence humans psychologically; brightness varies greatly (not simply on/off, light/dark) (Table 17.1)
B. Bright light found to suppress melatonin secretion from pineal gland in humans (about 1980)
C. As a result, bright light found to be successful in treatment of major depression that had seasonal pattern (fall/winter depressions)
D. Some applications of light therapy
  1. Seasonal affective disorder (SAD)
  2. Nonseasonal affective disorder (evening light if early morning awakening) or as augmentation to antidepressant

TABLE 17.1 Examples of Environmental Light Levels*	
Location/Time	Lux

Indoors

Home	200–500
Office	400–700
Drafting Room	500–1000

Outdoors (Spring Equinox)

Sunrise	6:10 a.m.	750
	6:20 a.m.	2500
	6:30 a.m.	5000
	6:45 a.m.	10,000
Noon	12:00	92,500
	5:30 p.m.	10,000
	5:45 p.m.	5000
	5:55 p.m.	2500
Sunset	6:10 p.m.	750

*Approximately middle U.S. latitude.

   3. Treatment of depression during pregnancy (to avoid medication use)
   4. Premenstrual dysphoric disorder
   5. Bulimia nervosa
   6. Jet lag
   7. Shift work adaptation
   8. Day/night abnormalities in Alzheimer's disease
   9. Advanced or delayed sleep phase disorders
   10. Adjusting from weekend schedule to work-week schedule
   11. Adjusting to daylight savings time
  E. Figure 17.1 shows optimal time for using light in selected applications
  F. May be primary treatment or adjunctive to medications
  G. *Brightness* of light used became key factor in efficacy rather than whether light was "full spectrum" (closest to mimicking the sunlight's color spectrum distribution), fluorescent, or incandescent

	Jet lag travel*	Daylight savings	Weekend ↔ work week adjustment	Depression type	**Light therapy given in**
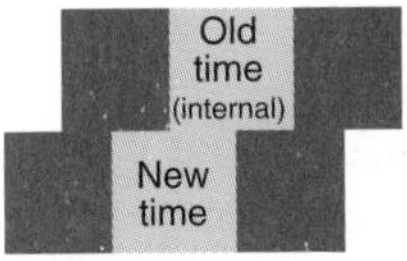 Old time (internal) / New time	East-ward	Spring 2 AM → 3 AM (clock ahead)	Sunday → Monday transition	SAD (atypical features)	**Morning** to advance rhythm
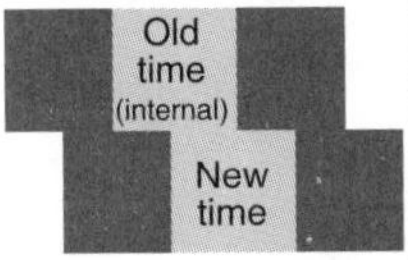 Old time (internal) / New time	West-ward	Fall 1 AM ← 2 AM (clock back)	Friday → Saturday transition (usually not a problem)	Typical depression and pre-menstrual dysphoric disorder (PMDD)	**Evening** to delay rhythm

*Depends upon number of time zones crossed

■ = Daylight

■ = Dark

FIGURE 17.1 Chronobiological conditions grouped by similarity.

H. Administration methods
  1. Natural means
    a. Exposing oneself to outdoor light at optimal times of day for effect
  2. Light devices
    a. Numerous types available; have not been compared regarding best efficacy
    b. Format
      i. Light boxes (manufactured by numerous companies)
        (1) Ultraviolet (UV) light is not as important for treatment of most symptoms of SAD, so it should be filtered out by these devices to reduce exposure to harmful effects of UV light
      ii. Incandescent bulbs of sufficient brightness
      iii. Light visor (although less definable dose-response relationship compared with other light sources)
      iv. Dawn simulator

(1) Gradually increasing brightness of light to patient at critical time of day-night cycle eliminates the need to either be awake or have the eyes open.

(2) The device simulates exposure to light earlier in the day as occurs in spring and summer.

I. Acute-phase treatment of seasonal depression (fall/winter type)

    1. Approximate dosing of light in seasonal depression is 10,000 lux for 30 minutes, 5000 lux for 1 hour, or 2500 lux for 2 hours, usually in the morning, but sometimes people do better with evening use of light

        a. For photographic light meters: one foot candle $\approx$ 10.76 lux

J. Maintenance of improvement

    1. Ideas on maintenance therapy vary, but some suggest on about 15 minutes per day

K. Prevention of seasonal depressive episode

    1. Begin light therapy 1 or 2 weeks before typical onset of symptoms

L. Light therapy can precipitate mania (like other antidepressant treatments); hence, follow same precautions in bipolar patients as with other antidepressant interventions

M. Patients are told not to stare at lights but to allow light to face the direction of their eyes while they may be doing other activities like reading or watching television

N. Mechanism of action

    1. Unknown; different theories

        a. Shift of circadian phase (e.g., morning light advances circadian rhythm in winter to be more like it is in summer)

        b. Photon theory (amount of light important regardless of time of day given)

 MENTOR TIPS DIGEST

- Advise your patients to write down important things that they want to remember that occur during acute phase ECT treatment.
- Memory impairments due to major depression *improve with ECT;* make sure to explain this anticipated benefit to your patient.

• Although low-dose bilateral ECT has slightly better efficacy than high-dose unilateral ECT, efficacy is close enough that clinically high-dose unilateral ECT is a good option for many patients sensitive to cognitive side effects of bilateral ECT.

Resources

www.UBCsad.ca
www.SLTBR.org
www.CET.org
   The above are all excellent Web sites on light therapy and seasonal affective disorder.

Chapter Self-Test Questions

Circle the correct answer. After you have responded to the questions, check your answers in Appendix A.

1. In electroconvulsive therapy, which of the following is most directly responsible for the therapeutic value of the treatment?
   a. Electrical stimulation
   b. Seizure
   c. Succinylcholine
   d. The psychological meaning of the procedure

2. Which of the following is similar in both electroconvulsive therapy and antidepressant medications?
   a. Down-regulation of beta-adrenergic receptors
   b. Equally therapeutic in major depression with psychotic features
   c. Equally therapeutic in mania
   d. Equal overall efficacy

3. During electroconvulsive therapy (ECT) a blood pressure cuff is inflated above systolic blood pressure on one arm (before succinylcholine is given) for which of the following reasons?
   a. Avoid succinylcholine falsely affecting blood pressure reading

b. To be able to confirm that a seizure occurred by motor movement of that extremity by seizure

c. To see if patient is awake

d. To speed up time required to administer ECT treatment

4. After acute phase treatment with electroconvulsive therapy, which of the following medication combinations has the best evidence regarding its ability to prevent recurrence of major depression?

a. Fluoxetine plus bupropion

b. Nortriptyline plus chlordiazepoxide

c. Nortriptyline plus lithium

d. Phenelzine plus chlorpromazine

5. Using currents to change electrical environment of targeted nerve or brain tissue to get desired effect is referred to as:

a. Neuroleptic.

b. Neuromodulation.

c. Neuropsychology.

d. Neurotoxicity.

 See the testbank CD for more self-test questions.

PART five

five

TREATMENT SETTINGS AND SUBSPECIALTIES

TREATMENT SETTINGS, SYSTEMS, AND OTHER CLINICAL ISSUES

18

**Michael R. Privitera, MD, MS, and
Jeffrey M. Lyness, MD**

I. Overview

A. This chapter deals with issues of where you will be working and with whom.

B. As a trainee, draw on core assessment skills in all sites, but learn how to focus your evaluations in relation to your setting.

C. As with any field of medicine, learn how to make a hierarchy in your mind as to what needs to be done first, next, and so forth.

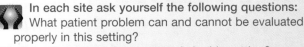

Because safety issues are always a priority, make sure that you, your patient, and others are safe before proceeding further. Do not be afraid to ask others for help or advice if concerns arise on safety.

D. Favored treatment modalities vary in relation to a setting's intended target patient population.
   1. Some treatments, such as group therapy aimed at specific problems (e.g., eating disorders, substance abuse), may work best when embedded in a larger treatment program.
E. Ideally, you will have a chance to work in multiple settings to get a better sense of breadth of psychiatry (although the length of your clinical rotation might preclude this). Define and refine your skills based on learning what techniques are used in all sites and which are limited to specific circumstances.

In each site ask yourself the following questions: What patient problem can and cannot be evaluated properly in this setting?
What are the patient outcome goals in this setting?
How does this setting relate to broader systems of psychiatric, medical, and other patient care?
What is the role of the psychiatrist and of other disciplines in achieving goals of this setting?

II. Treatment Settings
   A. Inpatient psychiatric units
      1. Overview
         a. May exist in general (i.e., medical-surgical) hospitals
         b. May be free-standing structures
            i. Privately owned
            ii. Publicly funded (e.g., state mental hospitals)
         c. Most serve general psychiatry population
         d. Programs to target specific patients (e.g., by age, diagnosis, or other commonality) may exist in general units or be sole offering of a subspecialty unit
      2. Short-term units
         a. Overview

    i. Classified such by average length of stay (LOS): e.g., short-term units may have LOS in days; long-term units may have LOS in weeks or months; partial hospital programs (PHPs) may have LOS in a brief number of weeks, whereas day treatment programs may have patients come for weeks or months

    ii. Are most common type of unit—many socioeconomic forces have made this so

    iii. Because fewer patients admitted than previously, those who are have *higher acuity level*

    iv. Differences in patient populations and treatment goals

b. Kind of care is oriented more toward *focused problem,* less toward diagnosis per se

    i. Focused problem to be identified requires careful psychiatric and medical evaluation and must be put in context of social environment of patient, including supports and stressors

> Example of focused problem versus overall disorder: patient's diagnosis may be major depression, but reason requiring admission is the *focused problem* of suicidal ideation. Once suicidal ideation is safe enough for outpatient care, patient would be discharged even though major depression is not fully remitted.

c. Treatments

    i. Somatic therapies (medications, electroconvulsive therapy [ECT] as appropriate)

    ii. Individual psychotherapy

      (1) "Here and now" issues

      (2) Psychoeducation (helping patient and family understand illness and treatment)

      (3) Crisis-oriented supportive psychotherapy

    iii. Group work or involvement in unit "milieu"

      (1) Highly structured task-oriented groups for patients at lower functioning (e.g., acutely psychotic or disorganized patients)

      (2) Talk-oriented therapy groups with focus on short-term issues for higher-functioning patients

      iv. Family work
        (1) Very important in most cases for:
          (A) Further data gathering
          (B) Aligning family support in patient's treatment and discharge plan
          (C) Providing psychoeducation and support to family
      v. Liaison with previous or future outpatient treaters, caregivers, or social agencies with aims of:
        (1) Data gathering
        (2) Psychoeducation
        (3) Solidification of discharge plan that provides for patient's needs
      vi. To accomplish preceding tasks rapidly requires coordinated efforts of multidisciplinary team
        (1) Psychiatrist is usual nominal team "captain" with ultimate responsibility for proper diagnosis and treatment plan implementation
        (2) Precise distribution of role responsibilities varies widely in different units and professional communities

3. Long-term units
  a. Overview
      i. Encompass variety of patient populations
      ii. Length of stay may be several weeks, months, or years
      iii. Less common, due to various socioeconomic forces
      iv. Patients typically admitted after failing many attempts at conventional therapies (may have included several short-term unit hospitalizations)
      v. Conditions: often marked by chronicity, treatment refractoriness, noncompliance, or several psychiatric or substance-abuse comorbidities
      vi. Tend to be *free-standing* rather than based in general hospitals
  b. Types
      i. Private long-term hospitals
        (1) Tend to have patients of higher socioeconomic strata — because health insurance plans often do not pay for these stays
        (2) Typical diagnostic groups
          (A) Intractable psychotic disorders such as schizophrenia

       (B) Severe personality disorders with comorbid mood, anxiety, or substance-use disorders

     (3) Some cater to specific diagnoses, e.g., severe and chronic eating disorders, post-traumatic stress disorder (PTSD)

  ii. Publicly funded long-term units

     (1) Serve many with few socioeconomic resources (which may contribute to, or be the result of, their psychopathology); (see later section on Systems of Care.)

     (2) Patients often have:

       (A) Chronic psychotic disorders (such as severe intractable schizophrenia or schizoaffective disorder).

       (B) Chronic or disabling mood disorders.

       (C) "Organic" mental disorders.

     (3) Patient populations vary by referral source (e.g., Veteran Affairs hospital units have many patients with combat related PTSD)

  iii. Long-term units in general

     (1) Often continue somatic therapies with more emphasis on more *intensive psychotherapies*

       (A) Rehabilitative (e.g., teaching social and vocational skills to patients with schizophrenia)

       (B) Exploratory psychodynamic or behavioral treatments—depending on patients served and traditions of institution

       (C) Intensive individual psychotherapy

       (D) Therapeutic milieu, with group therapies and activities forming major part of treatment plan

       (E) Longer-term family issues in ongoing family therapies

B. Partial hospital and day treatment programs (DTPs)

  1. PHPs

    a. Aim: treat acutely ill patients—often attempting to avert or shorten inpatient hospitalization

    b. Level of multidisciplinary staffing close to that of inpatient unit

    c. Often, full day's program 5 days per week

    d. Usually have a target or maximum length of stay (helps both patient and treatment team focus on achievable short-term goals)

   e. Free-standing or located in a general or psychiatric hospital
   f. Usually have close administrative or physical ties with inpatient units
   g. Usually emphasize group activities and therapies, but also close attention to somatic therapies and individual and family work
   h. Eligibility and diagnostic criteria similar to inpatient admissions but patients need to be safe enough—i.e., not imminently dangerous to themselves or others—to be able to go home at end of day
   i. Patients need means, desire, and motivation to come to program as staff cannot force them to attend
   j. Most programs open to general psychiatry patients, but some may be subspecialty-oriented
   2. DTPs
   a. Structurally less intensive versions of PHPs
   b. Lower staff-to-patient ratios, fewer psychiatrists (and general medical personnel) available
   c. Even more prominent role of groups than in PHPs
   d. Some or all patients come for shorter days or fewer days per week
   e. Clearly *less acute* than PHPs
   f. Goals more analogous to rehabilitative aims of long-term inpatient units
   g. Lower intensity but longer lengths of stay than in PHPs (many weeks to months) or indefinite "residence"
   h. Often serves as a *source of structure* that is useful to patient's improved functioning
   i. As a result of nature of patient's needs, such programs are often sub-specialized to better address specific needs of patients
 C. Outpatient settings
   1. Excellent opportunity for trainees, when possible, to see patients with major psychopathology in periods of relative symptomatic improvement
   2. Sources of variability
   a. *Site:* e.g., hospital-based clinic, free-standing private or public mental health clinic, private office, home visits ("house calls" are enjoying a minor resurgence in psychiatry as in general medicine)

b. *Practice staff structure:* e.g., solo psychiatrist, psychiatrist group (akin to models of group coverage in general medicine), multidisciplinary team
c. *Clinical problems encountered:* e.g., general psychiatric practice versus practice limited to certain diagnoses (mood disorders clinic) or specific treatment modalities (behavioral therapy center)
d. *Types of services offered:* e.g., consultation; crisis intervention; short-term or long-term psychotherapy; ongoing "medication management" without formal psychotherapy; individual, family, or group psychotherapies; most sites offer some combination of above, depending on clinical needs
e. *Length of patient visits:* e.g., quarter hour (brief follow-ups on known patients), half hour (lengthier follow-ups; some forms of psychotherapy with selected patients), hour (most traditional psychotherapies; first evaluation), longer visits (extensive evaluations; some crisis interventions)
f. *Frequency of patient visits:* e.g., weekly (most psychotherapies and acute illness management), two or more times per week (intensive exploratory long-term psychotherapy or psychoanalysis, severe acuity/crisis management), biweekly or even much less often (patients who are improving or stable for maintaining wellness)
g. *Availability of procedures* (e.g., physical evaluations from simple orthostatic vital-sign checks to full workups, phlebotomy, electrocardiograms, light therapy, outpatient ECT)
D. Consultation services
1. Overview
   a. Pathognomonic feature involves essence of psychiatrist's relationship to patient
      i. Most other circumstances *patient* is clearly person *being served,* and psychiatrist has ultimate responsibility to treat, educate, and otherwise intervene with patient
      ii. In consultation, *referring provider* is being primarily *served* (serving patient indirectly by using specialty expertise to answer referral questions as referring provider still has ultimate responsibility)
      iii. Enormously useful arrangement, but relationship can get somewhat less clear when consultant comes to assume some ongoing responsibility for patient's treatment

(1) Hence, important to make clear to patient and provider who has overall responsibility and authority for patient's care or what certain pieces of this responsibility may be delegated to expert consultants

2. Questions to consider
   a. *Who really wanted the consultation?*
      i. Usually straightforward: referring physician wanted consultation
      ii. Occasionally, official referring person is not primarily invested in consultation
         (1) May have been prompted by other providers (other consultants, residents, medical students, nursing staff), social workers (who may hope psychiatric consultation will expedite their efforts regarding patient disposition), patient's family, or patient
         (2) Understanding source of request will help you answer important questions following and help direct recommendations most helpfully
   b. *Now that you know who referred patient, what do you know about the referrer?*
      i. More you know about referrer, and more of an ongoing relationship you have with him/her, you are better able to figure out implicit questions of consult (see following)
      ii. What are relative strengths and limitations of person's knowledge and skills in psychiatric issues?
      iii. What are his or her attitudes toward mental disorders, psychiatry in general, you in particular?

> Some settings establish formal administrative structures linking psychiatric consultants with referrers, known as liaison arrangements. However, liaison-type work happens with all effective psychiatric consultation, creating frameworks and interpersonal relationships that make consultations more helpful to referrers and patients alike.

   c. *What is the explicit reason for consultation?*
      i. Extremely important to ask referrers to identify what it is they want you to do

(1) Sometimes request is vague: "I know patient has emotional distress, but I do not know what it is. Please do a diagnostic assessment."

(2) Dialogue between you and referrer may narrow focus
   (A) "Please evaluate this patient's suicidal ideation."
   (B) "Recommend an antidepressant." [After your evaluation, you may not agree patient needs an antidepressant]
   (C) "Evaluate patient's capacity to refuse medical treatment."
   (D) "Recommend treatment to reduce agitation."

d. *What are implicit reasons for consultation?*
   i. Asking this question means addressing *process* as well as *content* of consultation
   ii. Many times there are *no* implicit or hidden reasons for consultation; yet, important to look carefully for behind-the-scenes dynamics
   iii. When such reasons do arise, particularly with psychiatric issues, often quite affect-laden
   iv. Must be addressed tactfully to complete consultation satisfactorily
   v. Example: medical team asks in open-ended fashion to evaluate patient's capacity to refuse medical treatment
      (1) They likely have their own opinion (or sometimes mutually opposing opinions)
      (2) May have strong affects regarding this patient who is refusing their treatment
      (3) If your opinion differs from theirs or from what they expected you to indicate, careful explanation, discussion, and other liaison-type interactions may be needed to help team to accept your opinion and implement appropriate treatment plan; your discussion may also be helpful to team in resolving their own conflicts about case (which leads to better serving patient's interest)

3. Consultation settings
   a. *Inpatient hospital floors*
      i. Most common setting clinically as well as for academic/teaching consultation services

   b. *Outpatient primary care, specialty clinics, services* (e.g., dialysis units): "on site" (i.e., at clinic)
   c. *Outpatient psychiatric practices* (i.e., in psychiatrist's own office)
   d. *Residential settings* (e.g., nursing homes, adult care facilities, group homes)
   e. *Forensic settings* (e.g., prisons, court-related consultations, attorney- or insurance company–requested consultations related to legal actions or disability claims)
   f. *Employers* (companies may request consultation on individual basis for specific employee or group basis for more global occupational difficulties—this latter example more often performed by occupational psychologists)
E. Psychiatric emergency rooms
   1. Overview
   a. As with other emergency rooms (ERs), psychiatric emergency rooms' main functions are:
      i. Assess all comers
      ii. Initiate emergent-level treatments
      iii. Link up patients with appropriate subsequent services
         (1) Range: inpatient admissions, outpatient treatments, variety of other dispositions (including no treatment at all)
   b. Main psychiatric skills are diagnostic and situational assessment techniques
   c. Crisis interventions (medications, individual or family psychotherapies) are often employed to improve patient's clinical state and use least restrictive means of care (e.g., avoiding inpatient stay when possible)
   d. Unlike patients often encountered in other settings, some patients in ERs have never been diagnosed or treated psychiatrically

> As a trainee in "psych ER" (or "EW," "ED," or whatever your hospital calls it), you will have an opportunity to hone assessment and crisis intervention skills with an enormous range of patient diagnoses and problems. Thus, your clerkship is a wonderful exposure to broad clinical material.

2. Examples of types of problems and situations you may encounter
   a. True psychiatric emergencies: e.g., suicidal ideation, homicidal ideation
   b. Acute exacerbations of major mental disorders: acute psychosis; mania; severe depression, sometimes in course of comorbid Axis II disorders
   c. Substance use–related syndromes: intoxication; withdrawal; substance-induced mood; psychotic or other disorders; drug-seeking behavior, such as patients asking for pain medications or hypnotics
   d. New-onset psychiatric symptoms of major or less major proportions: all of preceding, plus anxiety and cognitive deficit syndromes (in less severe cases serves as diagnostic and triage center for outpatient care)
   e. Other secondary psychiatric syndromes (i.e., medical illnesses that present with prominent behavioral symptoms, leading to triage to psychiatric part of ER)
   f. Consultations to medical/surgical ER (e.g., problems that present a mixture of preceding, plus concerns previously discussed under consultation services)

III. Multidisciplinary Roles and Teams
A. Overview
   1. Private psychiatric practices may operate most often solely with psychiatrists, but other treatment settings are staffed by a variety of professionals.
   2. The roles of these professionals may vary from one setting to another and may overlap to some extent.
   3. To trainees new to psychiatry, this profusion of disciplines and roles may seem confusing, and the role of physician may seem less clear than in other medical specialties.
      a. However, psychiatric physicians do have well-defined roles in each setting, which will become apparent as you gain knowledge and experience in the field.
   4. You will find that other professionals have much to offer you in your educational experience.
   5. The following section briefly discusses backgrounds and roles of some of professionals you will encounter.

B. Psychiatrists

1. Physicians with specialty residency training in diagnosis and treatment of patients with mental disorders

2. Training: at least 4 years of residency after medical school

   a. PGY-I (internship) year consists of at least 4–6 months of medicine, pediatrics, or other nonpsychiatric services, with rest of year usually including neurology (2 months required before completing psychiatry residency) and psychiatry rotations; some programs make first year all nonpsychiatric medical services

   b. Remaining years

      i. Exposure to psychiatric inpatient, outpatient, ER, and consultation settings

      ii. Seminars cover wide range of basic and applied topics

      iii. Intensive one-to-one faculty-clinical supervision helps develop individual, family, and group psychotherapy abilities along with diagnostic and psychopharmacological skills

3. Psychotherapeutic skills are not unique (other professionals are able to deliver quality psychotherapy)

4. Specifically skilled regarding diagnosis (particularly in relation to medical illnesses that can be comorbid with, or contributory to, psychopathology) and development of biopsychosocial treatment plans, including somatic therapies

5. At most academic medical centers, psychiatrists are more or less "captains" of multidisciplinary treatment teams and have ultimate attending-level responsibility for patients

6. At other settings, psychiatrists play a consulting role to other mental health professionals who are primary treatment providers (sometimes this role is termed "medical backup," although many believe this phrase inappropriate depending on lines of responsibility at different institutions and sometimes from medicolegal perspective)

C. Psychologists

1. Some trained at master's degree level

   a. These persons are typically employed as psychotherapists either in private practice or in clinic or in other group multidisciplinary settings

2. Most psychologists in academic settings have doctorate-level training, either Ph.D. (doctor of philosophy) in psychology or Psy.D. (doctor of psychology) degree

  a. Clinical psychologists are the focus here: experimental psychologists do not see or treat patients but conduct research ranging from molecular biology to animal or human subject work

 3. Psy.D. training includes classroom and clinical work and strongly oriented toward developing skills and knowledge needed for clinical practice

 4. Ph.D. training includes classroom, clinical, and research experiences

  a. This education includes much deeper and broader exposure to basic sciences of psychology and research methodologies than most physicians obtain during their undergraduate or postgraduate medical training.

  b. This combination of psychological and methodological training makes psychologists qualified to interpret psychological testing (see Chapter 5).

 5. Clinical experiences of doctorate psychology trainees vary widely

  a. Some rotate through academic psychiatry settings and develop diagnostic and treatment planning analogous to, but not identical with, as they do not have the medical training as mentioned in psychiatrist section (e.g., more extensive education in psychological sciences but cannot diagnose or treat comorbid medical conditions, prescribe medications, or administer ECT)

  b. Others may not train in psychiatric settings but gain experience and skills in administering outpatient psychotherapies (individual, group, family) or using psychological skills in nonpatient settings (e.g., corporate psychology)

 6. May serve many roles in multidisciplinary psychiatric clinical settings

  a. Some roles—quite focused, such as providing psychotherapy or psychological testing

  b. Other roles—broader, including leading treatment teams, clinics, or units

D. Nurses

 1. Staff registered nurses

  a. In inpatient units, PHPs, and day treatment programs

   i. Responsible for management of overall milieu, including issues of patient safety (suicidal ideation and aggressivity)

    ii. Trained for careful observations of patients' behaviors and interpersonal interactions, using data to collaborate with other multidisciplinary treatment team members to help make diagnostic assessments, implement therapeutic interventions, and monitor patient response

    iii. May participate in family meetings

    iv. Lead unit groups

    v. Responsible for physical care assessments and interventions similar to nursing roles on general medical units

  2. Nurses with master's degree

    a. Have additional training in psychiatric diagnosis and psychotherapies

    b. May offer psychotherapy independently in private practice

    c. May evaluate and psychotherapeutically treat patients in multidisciplinary settings such as clinics

  3. Nurse practitioners

    a. Have additional training in diagnosis and therapeutics (including psychopharmacology)

    b. Have limited prescription privileges

    c. Can function with greater autonomy, again analogous to role of nurse practitioners in general medical settings

    d. Some go into private practice, having collaborative arrangement with psychiatrist

  4. Ph.D. in nursing

    a. Most often administrators or educators

E. Social workers

  1. In addition to standard training received by all social workers (including bachelor's, master's, or higher-level degrees), psychiatric social workers have additional educational experiences related to psychopathology and psychotherapies

  2. In multidisciplinary academic medical center settings, typically take a prominent role in involving families in patient's treatments

    a. This may include obtaining history from collateral informants, leading or co-leading family meetings that offer psychoeducation or other psychotherapeutic interventions

  3. May also lead unit groups

  4. Usually responsible for liaison with community agencies to access resources and implement optimal discharge planning (often after discussion with multidisciplinary team)

a. Often requires developing and maintaining relationships with relevant systems of care external to own unit

  5. In private practice, psychiatric social workers (especially those with master's-level or higher training) may offer wide variety of psychotherapies, including individual work; many have interests and practices tending to emphasize family or group therapies

F. Activities therapists

  1. Multidisciplinary treatment settings often employ persons with training in specialized fields such as recreational, art, music therapy

  2. Varied modalities used in groups or individual

    a. Designed to assess and develop psychosocial, cognitive, and physical skills important in rehabilitation from psychiatric illnesses

  3. May also lead other unit groups and work with members of treatment team to manage unit milieu and implement individualized patient treatment plans

  4. Some activities therapists may see patients privately for ongoing therapy

    a. Goals often analogous to goals of other longer-term psychotherapies, using modalities of art or music to facilitate expression of thoughts and affects, and serve as vehicle for development of therapeutic alliance with therapist

G. Therapists with other backgrounds

  1. Other kinds of psychotherapists (often with master's degree in counseling or education) or occupational or physical therapists: may aid usefully in assessment or treatment of psychiatric patients, particularly geriatric patients and severely and persistently mentally ill (SPMI) patients who need longer-term psychosocial rehabilitations

H. Paraprofessionals

  1. Psychiatric technicians ("psych techs") and nursing assistants may play prominent role in patient care, especially in acute hospital settings

  2. Educational backgrounds and work experience may vary, depending on requirements of employing institution

  3. Typically work closely with nursing staff to manage unit milieu, help implement psychiatric treatment plans, and provide needed physical care

IV. Systems of Care

A. "Traditional" and private insurance
  1. Fee for service, often with cap available
  2. No preauthorizations for care needed
  3. Most expensive premiums as pay-out risks from insurance companies not managed or controlled

B. Health maintenance organizations (HMOs)
  1. Patients may see only HMO-participating providers (psychiatrists, psychologists, psychiatric social workers, nurse practitioners, or master's-level nurses may be allowed on certain provider "panels").
  2. Only some HMOs have well-integrated system of care for patients in need of psychiatric services.
  3. Most have caps on mental health utilization.
     a. Maximum number of outpatient visits per year; maximum number of inpatient days per year (or per lifetime)
     b. Many HMOs use PHP days toward inpatient cap (e.g., ratios of 2 or 3 PHP days utilize 1 inpatient day from total yearly inpatient cap)
  4. Some use clinic model for outpatient visits, whereby patients primarily see less expensive non-physician therapists for intake or ongoing psychotherapy, with psychiatrists serving as backup consultation regarding medications, diagnostic issues, and shape of overall treatment plan.
  5. Most require preauthorization for specialist (e.g., psychiatric) care.
  6. Usually, the PCP is the "gatekeeper" to allow/not allow specialty services.
  7. HMOs clearly reduce mental health expenditures in the short run.
     a. Counterarguments:
        i. Quality and quantity of care considerably less than ideal
        ii. Cost savings may be illusory, because patients with untreated or poorly treated mental disorders have higher utilization of general medical resources
        iii. Most HMO systems tend not to be geared toward patients with severe, debilitating mental disorders

C. SPMI
  1. Includes persons with chronic psychotic disorders (primarily schizophrenia) along with malignant, treatment-refractory, debilitating forms of mood, personality, and other disorders

2. By definition, persons tend to have high rates of psychiatric hospitalization; need highly structured, intensive, long-term psychiatric treatments and psychosocial rehabilitation
3. Systems of care for this population must include access to inpatient units, short-term and long-term PHPs and DTPs, clinics, and wide array of ancillary services (including social work, occupational and activities therapies, vocational rehabilitation, and others)
4. Intensive case managers (ICMs): strategy to help low-volume, high-intensity caseloads to be more compliant with medications and provider appointments, meals, transportation, or other needs—goal of successfully keeping patient in most independent living environments possible
5. Wide range of intensive services is expensive
   a. Much of frontline care provided by non-physician (i.e., less expensive) professionals
   b. Psychiatrists usually conduct diagnostic evaluations at intake; initiate and monitor somatic therapies; supervise treatment plans, including progress of psychosocial therapies
   c. Patients usually too impaired to hold down steady jobs to have private health insurance; thus largely depend on public support
      i. Support includes federal and state monies (through programs like Medicaid)
      ii. Distribution mostly at state level—current SPMI systems thematically (and sometimes literally) direct descendant of days when huge state hospitals housed many thousands of chronically ill psychiatric patients
      iii. In principle, money that used to pay for long-term inpatient care has been shifted to provide such current services
D. Substance dependence
   1. Programs exist in universe parallel to rest of mental health services
   2. Numerous points of intersection with psychiatry universe but autonomous domain nonetheless
   3. Provide for safe management of acute withdrawal from alcohol and other drugs (detox)
   4. Inpatient, PHPs, DTPs and traditional outpatient models of treating drug dependency

5. Many extrinsic factors including historical development of addiction treatment separate from insane asylums, payment mechanisms play role in separation of systems

6. Intrinsic factors, such as treatment methods, differ: e.g., harsher, more confrontational styles that assume patients may be untruthful about their substance use permeate substance-dependence treatment—somewhat antithetical to traditional spirit or practice of rest of psychiatry

7. High comorbidity of substance-dependence and SPMI patients led to blending approach for such patients to be more successful than either separately when both problems exist; such "dually diagnosed," or mentally ill chemical abusers (MICA), patients now can get help in most SPMI programs that have developed MICA services

8. Many self-help (not professionally run)

9. Alcoholics Anonymous, Narcotics Anonymous, and various other 12-step programs exist in abundance in most American communities and are effective in helping to achieve and maintain sobriety—sometimes used in combination with professional resources

E. Mental retardation/developmental disabilities

1. Public funds support educational and residential care needs of people with significant mental retardation or developmental disabilities (MRDD), such as autism

2. Although defined in DSM-IV as mental disorders, combination of historical, financial, and clinical issues resulted in system separate from traditional child and adult psychiatric treatment systems

3. Other psychiatric symptoms (e.g., depression, psychosis) and behavioral disturbances (e.g., self-injurious actions, aggressivity) frequently coexist with MRDD

   a. Treatable in traditional psychiatric settings in patients with borderline intellectual functioning (IQ 71–84 range) or mild mental retardation (IQ 50–55 up to 70)

   b. Those with more severe MRDD-spectrum illness, care is usually best provided by ongoing psychiatric consultation-liaison to MRDD facilities within which patient lives or works

F. Nursing homes and other geriatric care

1. Chapter 19 section on geriatric psychiatry discusses psychiatric issues in elderly at somewhat greater length

2. Chronic debilitating mental disorders, including psychiatric disturbances associated with dementing illnesses such as Alzheimer's disease, quite common in older persons

3. In decades past, many of most behaviorally disturbed demented elderly resided in state mental institutions; in recent years, deinstitutionalization has drastically shrunk number of such patients in state hospitals

  a. As result, many now cared for at home or in residencies originally designed for physically disabled such as nursing homes and adult care facilities (facilities have become de facto state hospital system for chronically mentally ill elderly)

  b. Psychiatric consultation/liaison services are required to successfully address such patients' needs in these settings

V. Legal and Ethical Issues in Psychiatry

A. Competency, capacity, and informed consent

  1. In the United States, people are presumed to be able to exercise their rights as citizens unless proven otherwise; therefore competency is presumed.

  2. It takes legal proceedings, including a judge's decision, to declare a person "incompetent" and take appropriate action, such as assigning legal guardianship.

  3. Physicians cannot determine *competency*. Physicians can offer an expert opinion as to whether a person has a mental disorder that is affecting his or her ability to perform a particular act such as making decisions regarding medical treatment; e.g., does a person have mental ability or decision-making *capacity* (DMC) to make such decisions to have adequate informed consent for decision?

    a. Three exceptions to informed consent:

       i. **Emergency treatment:** emergency must be serious and urgent

       ii. **Therapeutic privilege:** (rarely used as need to justify that patient could not psychologically withstand being informed of proposed treatment)

       iii. Competent patient **waives right** for information.

  4. Distinguish "bad decisions" and *free will* from lack of DMC.

> A useful example of a "bad decision" is a patient with alcoholism with cirrhosis of the liver who, although sober and having DMC, decides to continue to drink alcohol when he leaves the hospital.

5. Most determinations of DMC never reach the courts (nor should they) to determine legal competency.
6. Physicians must **estimate the likelihood** that a **court** would find the patient incompetent on basis of capacities demonstrated.
7. If estimated that a patient is likely to be found "incompetent," then engage mechanisms for obtaining a substitute decision (technically, obtain decision from health care proxy [HCP] or guardian who has authority to consent—unless emergency exception applies).
8. Capacity is both time- and issue-specific and is affected by severity of potential outcome and context of setting.
   a. Time: capacity may change over time (e.g., delirious patient when improves is expected to regain DMC, but in dementia with expected progressive decline it is unlikely that patient would regain DMC)
   b. Issue: therefore, capacity to do what?; for example, a delusional patient may not be able to decide whether to take medications recommended as he falsely believes doctor is trying to poison him; yet, the same patient may be able to fully manage his finances
   c. Potential outcome: if severe, would need to examine more closely and have a higher threshold for DMC; for example, a patient who is homeless, suffering from schizophrenia, having end-stage renal failure requiring dialysis, and wanting to leave against medical advice (AMA) would have a higher level of scrutiny than a homeless patient with schizophrenia who has pneumonia, has completed all but 1 day's treatment of antibiotics, and wants to leave AMA and says will take medicine as outpatient
   d. *Context of setting:* are there people around to help, or does patient live alone?; for example, elderly man with dementia who lives alone would have a higher threshold for DMC about discharge than an elderly man with dementia who would be living with his functional wife
9. *Criteria questions:* Do patients understand relevant information? Do they appreciate situation and its potential consequences? Can they make a reasoned decision? Do they communicate a choice?
10. Table 18.1 shows criteria for determining capacity and issues that may affect each criterion.

TABLE 18.1	
Criteria in Determining Capacity (XIX 5)	
Criteria*	**Issues Involved**
Understanding relevant information	Can be affected by deficits in attention, intelligence, memory (of words, phrases, ideas, and sequences of information; reception, storage, and retrieval); must comprehend fundamental meaning
Appreciating the situation and its consequences	Can understand what is told, without understanding specific implications that it carries for one's future; one must appreciate the illness,[†] consequences of treatment or its refusal, and likelihood of consequences
Making a reasoned decision	One must also demonstrate reasoning about the information and its consequences, comparing the benefits and risks of various treatment options in a logical way, consistent with one's values, to arrive at a decision
Communicating a choice	Can be affected by impairment of consciousness, thought disorder, disruption of short-term memory, and severe ambivalence.

*In all cases when evaluating the patient for decision-making capacity, make every effort to help the patient perform their best.

[†]Denial of illness can render a patient incompetent to render treatment decisions (*Guardianship of John Roe,* 411 Mass. 666, 670 [1992]).

11. Following are common ways that psychiatric symptoms may affect capacity.
   a. *Psychosis:* delusions may affect understanding or reasoning through medical circumstances or cause patient to be too distracted to process information appropriately
   b. *Depression:* some moderate to severe states of depression may impair DMC due to wish to die, hopelessness, nihilism, or guilt refusing needed care

   c. *Cognitive deficits:* delirious, demented, or amnestic patients may not comprehend or remember facts relevant to decision to manipulate information appropriately; lack of abstraction or frontal executive function impairments may affect reasoned DMC

12. Informed consent has the following features.

   a. It is responsibility of provider to give explanation of all necessary facts of condition, reasonable risks, benefits, and alternatives to proposed treatment (to promote rational decision making by patient)

   b. Patient would need to understand preceding factors to have capacity to provide such consent

B. Civil commitment

1. Clinically, many patients in acute phases of severe mental disorders will benefit from inpatient treatment.

2. For some, inpatient treatment may be the only alternative for clinical improvement, or it may be life-saving by preventing harm to themselves or others.

3. Sometimes patients do not want to be hospitalized due to very poor insight into their symptoms affecting their capacity to make decision to be hospitalized.

4. Well-intentioned clinicians may wish such incapacitated patients to be hospitalized against their will if necessary to receive proper care.

5. From legal perspective, the idea parallels the principles of *parens patriae* (government has obligations toward citizens unable to care for themselves) and *police powers* (government may protect its citizens from harming one another as in physical assaultiveness of some acutely mentally ill patients).

   a. These two principles underlie legal process of *civil commitment,* a specified mechanism that allows for involuntary psychiatric hospitalization of *certain* acutely ill patients. They must be an imminent risk to themselves (sometimes the principle may be extended to include inability to care for themselves) or others.

   b. These principles must always be balanced against the constitutional guarantee of liberty (which is why states provide legal representation to psychiatric patients to ensure *due process* is followed for those who want to contest physician's decision).

c. These mental hygiene statutes allow physicians (it may take more than one) to admit patients involuntarily.

d. Many states also have statutes that formalize status and rights of patients who *voluntarily* are admitted to psychiatric facilities.

C. Involuntary medication

1. Clinically, it may make little sense to hospitalize an acutely ill, dangerous, capacity-lacking patient and then allow the patient to refuse medications or other treatments needed to treat the acute state.

2. Legally however, involuntary treatment is an issue separate from commitment and can be considered a form of battery if medications are given over objections in a *non-emergent* setting (some states may not even allow emergent medications).

3. Most local jurisdictions have guidelines—statutes or local standards of practice—about how to handle involuntary medication situations for patients thought to lack capacity to refuse medication.

a. Local jurisdictions determine how much of these decisions are left to physicians (if any—depending on the state) and when courts need to be involved.

 MENTOR TIPS DIGEST

- Because safety issues are always priority, make sure that you, your patient and others are safe before proceeding further. Do not be afraid to ask others for help or advice if concerns arise on safety.
- In each site ask yourself the following questions: What patient problem can and cannot be evaluated properly in this setting?
  What are the patient outcome goals in this setting?
  How does this setting relate to broader systems of psychiatric, medical, and other patient care?
  What is the role of the psychiatrist and of other disciplines in achieving goals of this setting?
- Example of focused problem versus overall disorder: patient's diagnosis may be major depression, but reason requiring admission is the *focused problem* of

suicidal ideation. Once suicidal ideation is safe enough for outpatient care, patient would be discharged even though major depression is not fully resolved.

- Some settings establish formal administrative structures linking psychiatric consultants with referrers, known as liaison arrangements. However, liaison-type work happens with all effective psychiatric consultation, creating frameworks and interpersonal relationships that make consultations more helpful to referrers and patients alike.
- As a trainee in "psych ER" (or "EW," "ED," or whatever your hospital calls it), you will have an opportunity to hone assessment and crisis intervention skills with an enormous range of patient diagnoses and problems. Thus, your clerkship is a wonderful exposure to broad clinical material.
- A useful example of a "bad decision" is a patient with alcoholism with cirrhosis of the liver who, although sober and having DMC, decides to continue to drink alcohol when he leaves the hospital.

Resources

Appelbaum PS, Grisso T: Assessing patients' capacities to consent to treatment. N England Journal of Medicine 319:1635–1638, 1988.

Lyness JM: End-of-life care: Issues relevant to the geriatric psychiatrist. American Journal of Geriatric Psychiatry 12:457–472, 2004.

Chapter Self-Test Questions

Circle the correct answer. After you have responded to the questions, check your answers in Appendix A.

1. Which of the following is the primary classification mechanism for terming a unit "short-term unit"?

    a. Acuity level

    b. Average length of stay

   c. Staff-to-patient ratios

   d. Type of patient treated

2. Which of the following is more associated with day treatment programs compared with partial hospital programs?

   a. Acutely ill patients

   b. General psychiatric patients

   c. Long lengths of stay

   d. Somatic therapies

3. In consultation services, which of the following is most likely to be considered the "customer to be served"?

   a. Family member of patient

   b. Friend of patient

   c. Patient

   d. Referring provider

4. Which of the following mental health specialists has 4 years of residency training after medical school?

   a. Ph.D. nursing

   b. Psychiatric social worker

   c. Psychiatrist

   d. Psychologist

See the testbank CD for more self-test questions.

PSYCHIATRIC SUBSPECIALTIES

Michael R. Privitera, MD, MS, and Jeffrey M. Lyness, MD

I. Overview

A. Major psychiatric subspecialties are presented in this chapter.

B. Subspecialty fields developed because of special needs of certain subpopulations of psychiatric patients.

C. American Board of Psychiatry and Neurology (ABPN) offers subspecialty certification in these areas after demonstration of experience, training, and successfully passing ABPN board examinations.

D. The oldest ABPN subspecialty is Child and Adolescent Psychiatry.

II. Addiction Psychiatry

A. Focuses on evaluation and treatment of patients with drug, alcohol, and other substance-use disorders; those patients with dual diagnoses of substance-related disorders and other psychiatric disorders are well served by this subspecialty—mentally ill chemical abusers (MICAs)

B. Frequent clinical issues involved

    1. Detoxification and acute treatment of patients with substance-use and substance-induced disorders

    2. Use of psychoactive medications in treatment of psychiatric disorders that often accompany use of drugs

    3. Techniques for confrontation and intervention with substance abuser and dealing with defense mechanisms

    4. Psychological and social problems, medical and psychiatric disorders that often accompany use and abuse of drugs

    5. Psychotherapeutic modalities involved in management of substance-abusing patient, including individual, family, couples, and group therapy

III. Child and Adolescent Psychiatry

A. Medical specialty encompassing diagnosis and treatment of mental disorders in infants, children, and adolescents

B. Considerable overlap with practice of general (and other subspecialty) pediatrics and adolescent medicine

C. Numerous areas of commonality of perspective and practice with general psychiatry, as exemplified by training requirements

    1. 3 years of general psychiatry residency and 2 years of child psychiatry fellowship must be completed

D. Compared with general psychiatry, numerous differences in content and process of child psychiatry

> It is important to understand an overview of the differences between child and general psychiatry rotations for those who (by choice or assignment) train in child psychiatry settings.

    1. Developmental issues `XVII 1-2`

        a. Attention to these issues prominent in psychiatry and all biopsychosocially sophisticated medical care

        b. Obviously an inherent part of working with children

        c. Biological, psychological, and social changes over time in this population are rapid and profound

        d. Children's capabilities and limitations at each level of conceptual organization are quite different (not only from those of adults but also from those of pre-adults of different ages)

        e. Developmental issues inform everything—differential diagnosis, psychodynamic formulation, interviewing techniques, and treatment planning and implementation—and underlie remaining points in this section

    2. Family `XVII 2`

        a. Children are dependent on their families to greater extent than are most adults

        b. Assessment of child's family crucial to almost all child psychiatric evaluations

        c. Active involvement of family is usually at least important adjunct and can be primary or sole treatment modality

3. Social systems

    a. Nonfamily social systems are often crucial to assessment, management, and (for severe cases) placement of child psychiatry patients

    b. May include schools and other educational agencies, workshops and other vocational centers, residential facilities, and child protective services

4. Disorders that are more common in childhood

    a. Number of mental disorders in DSM-IV-TR are "usually first diagnosed in infancy, childhood, or adolescence"

       i. Mental Retardation **XVII 6**

          (1) Cognitive impairment with onset before 18 years

          (2) Broad continuum of severity, so specifiers (e.g., "mild") are used based on intelligence testing

      ii. Pervasive Developmental Disorders

          (1) Manifested by difficulties in several areas of development, unrelated to intellectual deficits

          (2) Include problems in social interactions, communication skills, and stereotypes

          (3) Autism probably best known; other examples include Rett's and Asperger's disorders **XVII 7**

      iii. Attention-Deficit/Hyperactivity Disorder (ADHD) **XVII 5**

          (1) Characterized by inattention along with impulsivity or motor hyperactivity

          (2) Lay press and some antipsychiatry (or antipsychopharmacology) organizations frequently point out difficulties distinguishing "normal" from abnormal symptoms and the reality that diagnosis can be difficult in some cases

 In ADHD cases, as in all areas of medicine, keep your clinical wits about you and balance risks versus benefits to the patient.

          (3) ADHD can be enormously impairing condition

          (4) Treatments (including psychotropics) can be quite helpful, often leading to substantial improvement in school or social performance

      iv. Tic Disorders

          (1) Tics are sudden, rapid, recurrent, nonrhythmic, stereotyped, involuntary motor movements or vocalizations.

(2) Motor tics are as simple as eye blinking or grimacing and include more complex behaviors such as jumping, touching, and grooming activities.

(3) Vocal tics range from sniffing or throat clearing to verbal utterances including coprolalia (use of obscene or otherwise inappropriate words).

(4) Tics may be secondary to a variety of substances and medical/neurological conditions.

(5) Tic disorder is diagnosed if tics are idiopathic.

(6) Diagnostic categories are defined by transience or chronicity and presence of motor or vocal tics.

(7) Tourette's disorder is defined by multiple motor tics *and* one or more vocal tics over a period of a year or more.

b. Other disorders

  i. Learning disorders

  ii. Communication disorders (expression or reception of language)

  iii. Conduct disorder (pervasive pattern of disruptive, dishonest, or aggressive behaviors; often precursor of antisocial personality disorder in adulthood) **XVII 5**

  iv. Oppositional defiant disorder (may be a precursor of conduct disorder)

  v. Feeding or eating disorders of infancy or early childhood (e.g., pica)

  vi. Elimination disorders (e.g., enuresis)

  vii. Separation anxiety disorder (relatively common; may develop in relation to life stress or significant loss — may be precursor of anxiety or mood disorders in adulthood)

5. Disorders presenting differently in childhood

  a. Most major disorders of adulthood (including psychotic, mood, anxiety, and somatoform disorders) may present during childhood but may or may not have different demographic or clinical characteristics in children

  b. Following are examples of potential differences **XVII 1**

    i. Schizophrenia

      (1) Uncommon in children, although prevalence in adolescents approaches that of adults (peak incidence is late teens to early twenties)

    (2) Children may manifest social withdrawal or eccentricities as prodrome (schizophrenia may be suspected but not confirmed until psychotic symptoms emerge, as depression or other behavioral conditions are in differential diagnosis)

    (3) Childhood schizophrenia must meet same diagnostic criteria as for adults, except role dysfunction criteria may be met by failure to achieve age-appropriate developmental advances rather than actual decline

  ii. Depression

    (1) The incidence and prevalence of major depression in children have been increasing, although some of apparent increase may result from attitudinal changes leading to greater recognition of illness and willingness to treat it by families and providers.

    (2) Criteria are the same as for adults, but role dysfunction may manifest as failure to achieve normal developmental goals.

    (3) In practice, children are less likely overtly to manifest classic mood and ideational symptoms of depression as spontaneously exhibiting or complaining of sad mood, guilt, or hopelessness.

    (4) The main overt indicators of depression in children include irritability, boredom or disinterest, somatization, social withdrawal, and "acting out" behaviors.

6. Therapeutics

  a. Crucial role of family therapy in treatment of children or adolescents

  b. Interventions with and by social agencies such as schools may be large part of strategies

  c. Individual diagnostic and psychotherapeutic sessions often organized around playing with toys, drawing, or other task-oriented activities to allow patients to express feelings and thoughts they might be able to access solely by face-to-face verbal contact

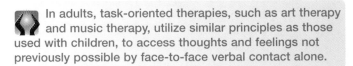
In adults, task-oriented therapies, such as art therapy and music therapy, utilize similar principles as those used with children, to access thoughts and feelings not previously possible by face-to-face verbal contact alone.

   d. Face-to-face talk therapy used as appropriate and tolerated,
      particularly with older children and adolescents
   e. Pharmacotherapy useful adjunct for many children, although
      is primary treatment far less often than in adult psychiatry
      i. Basic principles of drug use in children are the same as for
         adults, including careful attention to diagnosis and target
         symptoms.
      ii. Unfortunately, patient, family, and societal attitudes
         toward psychotropic medications for children may be even
         more negative than for adults.

IV. Forensic Psychiatry

   A. Application of psychiatric knowledge to legal matters
   B. Types of law include civil, criminal, and administrative
   C. May include evaluation and treatment of individuals so involved
      with the legal system
   D. Outpatient, inpatient forensic hospitals and jails common sites of
      practice
   E. Typical issues addressed include criminal culpability, insanity
      defense, competency evaluations to assist in defense, evaluation of
      malingering, determining risk of violence to self or others,
      disability evaluations, and treatment of patients who have
      interrelationships with the legal system
   F. Many have completed forensic psychiatry fellowship and have
      subspecialty board certification

V. Geriatric Psychiatry

   A. Overview
      1. Successful practice of psychiatry with older patients requires
         thorough grounding in general psychiatry, with specific
         expertise regarding mental disorders most common in
         later life
      2. Some amount of knowledge of and comfort with geriatric
         medicine, neurology, and gerontology important
      3. A recognized board subspecialty
      4. Fellowships in geriatric psychiatry available in multiple sites
         across the country
   B. Developmental issues
      1. Prominent developmental issues of later life underlie/overlay
         clinical work with older patients

2. Many issues relate to losses, including deaths, retirement, social isolation, and medical illnesses or functional disability in oneself and others ⟨VIII 10⟩

3. Biggest loss-related issue in aging is need to prepare psychologically for one's own death

   a. People (at various levels of explicitness) perform "life review," reexamination of life's past events and meanings

4. Aging is *not* all about loss

   a. Growing attention being paid to creativity and resiliency with aging

C. Family

   1. Older persons often closely engaged with, or dependent on, family members or other persons close to them as friends or neighbors

   2. As in child psychiatry, contact with family essential to full psychiatric assessment

   3. In case of elderly, "family" often means adult children or grandchildren as well as spouse

   4. Treatments often involve family as adjunctive or primary modality

D. Social systems

   1. As in child psychiatry, assessment and treatment of older persons may involve a variety of agencies or social systems, including home health aides and visiting nurse services; a range of alternative housing options, from senior independent apartments to adult homes that provide greater supervision to nursing homes that can provide skilled nursing care; psychiatric or dementia-oriented day programs; senior centers; Meals-on-Wheels programs; transportation services; and adult protective services.

E. Common new-onset psychiatric disorders in older persons

   1. Depressions (major depressions and variety of so-called "subsyndromal" states of clinically meaningful depressive symptoms that do not quite meet criteria for major depression)

   2. Dementia

   3. Delirium

   4. Psychoses (most due to preceding three categories; some due to delusional disorders or fuller panoply of symptoms consistent with schizophrenia criteria)

   5. Secondary syndromes (see "Comorbidity" following)

   6. Other (including adjustment disorders and alcohol dependence)

a. New-onset primary anxiety disorders and somatoform disorders are relatively uncommon in the elderly, although anxiety and somatoform symptoms may be common with above diagnoses, and some people with chronic anxiety, somatoform, or substance use disorders beginning earlier in life may still be symptomatic and need treatment in their later years.

F. Comorbidity
 1. In younger adults, psychiatric comorbidity common; e.g., mood and substance use disorders existing simultaneously, each contributing to the other, making treatment more complicated and prognosis not as good
 2. In elderly, *medical* comorbidity is rule
    a. Declining physical health common with age
 3. Systemic or neurological conditions of older age often contribute to onset and course of late-life psychopathology either directly (e.g., intrinsic brain disease like Alzheimer's, systemic conditions that affect brain functioning) or as stressor affecting person's sense of self, family, other role functions
 4. DSM-IV-TR dichotomy between "primary" and "secondary" psychiatric syndromes seems particularly arbitrary and problematic in elderly
 5. Practice suggestions in care of elderly
    a. Maintain high level of suspicion for medical contributors when presented with new or worsened psychopathology
    b. Maintain high level of suspicion for psychiatric manifestations of medical illnesses, psychiatric contributions to somatic symptoms, frequent calls or office visits, noncompliance
    c. Aggressively target and treat all potentially treatable psychiatric syndromes and medical conditions, recognizing their frequent interrelationships

G. Therapeutics
 1. Family work in psychotherapy important in elderly population
 2. Group work can be viewed as useful
 3. Individual psychotherapy may be viewed with more stigma by older persons but may change as Baby-Boomers age
    a. Geriatric patients who do accept referral for individual work often ally well with their therapists and can benefit greatly from flexible supportive/expressive approaches as well as from focused evidence-based psychotherapies.

   4. Pharmacotherapy in elderly has several complicating factors `XVIII 3`
      a. Changes in drug absorption and metabolism, related to age or diseases associated with age, means lower doses may be needed to reach a given blood level
      b. Age-related changes in neurotransmitter activity make older brain more sensitive to central nervous system (CNS) side effects of psychotropics (including tremor, ataxia, dysarthria, sedation, delirium)
         i. Especially true if frank neurological disease
      c. Variability increases with age, so extent to which above two points are true varies astonishingly in different older persons
      d. Most published drug research used relatively healthy or younger subjects; treatment of elders with neurological or substantial systemic comorbidity often based on extrapolation from data obtained from other populations or based on anecdotal evidence

H. Suicide in elderly
   1. Older persons have highest suicide rates `XVIII 2`
   2. Older suicidal persons, as compared with younger persons, more likely to intend to die and use methods of greater lethality
   3. Of elderly who do kill themselves, most have diagnosable depressive disorder at time of death
      a. Rarely have they seen a mental health professional, but most saw their primary care provider within a few weeks of their suicide; therefore, public health efforts to reduce this significant cause of death in later life begin with improved recognition and treatment of depression in primary care settings.

VI. Pain Medicine
   A. Field diverse in scope; membership from such specialties as anesthesiology, internal medicine, neurology, neurological surgery, orthopedic surgery, physiatry, psychiatry
   B. As a subspecialty of ABPN, typically from psychiatrically, neurologically, or child-neurologically trained origins and offers certification in this area
   C. Patient population served includes acute, chronic, and cancer pain patients
   D. Primary or consultative care provided in ambulatory or hospital settings

VII. Psychosomatic Medicine (PSM) [Consultation-Liaison (C-L) Psychiatry]
  A. Newly recognized subspecialty of psychiatry, with first board certification examination offered in 2005
  B. "Psychosomatic medicine" new term recognized by ABPN for field of C-L Psychiatry
  C. In 1934 Rockefeller Foundation made grants to five universities to start psychiatric liaison departments to interface with medicine and surgery units
  D. As field, sub-specializes in consultative or concomitant care for diagnosis and treatment of psychiatric disorders and symptoms in medical, surgical, neurological, obstetrical patients
  E. Core difference of *consultative* role is that, technically, the "customer" is the service requesting consultation, not patient; yet, your interventions assist care of patient through primary team
  F. As prevalence of medical illness increases with age, many core concepts from field of Geriatric Psychiatry embedded in C-L Psychiatry
  G. Categories of problems commonly encountered by C-L Psychiatry
    1. Psychiatric presentations of medical conditions
    2. Medical presentations of psychiatric conditions
    3. Psychiatric reactions to medical conditions
    4. Psychiatric complications of medical conditions or treatments
    5. Medical complications of psychiatric conditions or treatments
    6. Comorbid medical and psychiatric conditions
    7. Combinations of preceding
  H. *Liaison* services occur by building professional relationships (administratively formal or informal) with various medical/surgical services, such as infectious disease (e.g., HIV-infected patients), cardiology (e.g., post-MI cases of depression), neurology (e.g., epilepsy, stroke, multiple sclerosis), obstetrical (e.g., high-risk pregnancy)
  I. As student rotation on C-L, there may be more opportunity for medical/psychiatric differential diagnosis and possibly less on opportunity to see effects of interventions over time, compared with colleagues on inpatient psychiatry; nonetheless, some patients seen on C-L are medically hospitalized for long periods; thus, opportunities to see effects of interventions

MENTOR TIPS DIGEST

• It is important to understand an overview of the differences between child and general psychiatry rotations for those who (by choice or assignment) train in child psychiatry settings.
• In ADHD cases, as in all areas of medicine, keep your clinical wits about you and balance risks versus benefits to the patient.
• In adults, task-oriented therapies, such as art therapy and music therapy, utilize similar principles as those used with children, to access thoughts and feelings not previously possible by face-to-face verbal contact alone.

Chapter Self-Test Questions

Circle the correct answer. After you have responded to the questions, check your answers in Appendix A.

1. Which of the following is the oldest formally recognized subspecialty of psychiatry?
   a. Addiction Psychiatry
   b. Child and Adolescent Psychiatry
   c. Geriatric Psychiatry
   d. Psychosomatic Medicine

2. Which of the following subspecialties of psychiatry focus on MICA patients?
   a. Addiction Psychiatry
   b. Child and Adolescent Psychiatry
   c. Geriatric Psychiatry
   d. Psychosomatic Medicine

 See the testbank CD for more self-test questions.

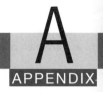

APPENDIX

ANSWERS TO SELF-TEST QUESTIONS

Below are the answers to the self-test questions that appear at the end of each chapter.

Part I: Psychiatry as a Field of Medicine

Chapter 1: Introduction to Psychiatry

1. b.

Response: Primary care has been referred to as "the de facto mental health system" because of the predominance of care being provided in the primary care provider setting.

2. d.

Response: The inability to describe or recognize one's own emotions (alexithymia) has been thought to be the mechanism by which emotional expression its unconsciously translated into somatic sensations.

3. a.

Response: Countertransference is important to recognize and manage so it does not interfere with more objective decision making on what treatment is best for the patient.

Chapter 2: Perspectives on Human Behavior

1. a.

Response: Different theories of human behavior provide different approaches that may be helpful in the care of a patient, each theory making its own unique contribution.

2. a.

Response: Bipolar Disorder is largely genetic; Major Depression is strongly genetic. In Personality Disorders and PTSD, genetic factors play a more distant role.

3. a.

Response: Aldosterone affects electrolytes. Female reproductive hormones may play a role in the predisposed individual. The HPA axis is hyperactive in Major Depression. Thyroid function is a primary disease that may overlap in symptoms with Mood Disorder and anxiety states. Thyroid hormone triiodothyronine has a direct pharmacological effect.

4. c.

Response: MRI shows higher resolution and hence more detail than CT.

5. b.

Response: Dopamine, norepinephrine, and serotonin have been extensively studied in psychiatric disorders. Glycine is an amino acid neurotransmitter that has not been closely linked to the pathophysiology of psychiatric disorders.

Part II: Psychiatric Workup

Chapter 3: History and Physical Examination

1. c.

Response: The patient's words on most prominent reasons for presentation are placed in the Chief Complaint section.

2. b.

Response: Psychiatric illness, like all medical illness, is confidential and considered protected health information (PHI). Access to PHI must be allowed by the patient or an appropriate representative of the patient.

3. d.

Response: Syndromic method of organization of the HPI implies having an overarching concept of the illness.

4. a.

Response: Having an overarching concept of the patient's illness drives the pertinence of information to the history.

5. c.

Response: Recent onset illness has no previous existence. Hence, all description of symptoms of illness is relevant to this recent illness only.

Chapter 4: Mental Status Examination

1. c.

Response: Categories of data are set forth in the MSE just as categories of data are set forth in the physical examination.

2. a.

Response: Large amounts of data can be obtained in any patient interview once the physician is trained to look for it.

3. a.

Response: Eye contact indicates connectivity to the interviewer.

4. d.

Response: Adventitious is defined as "outside," i.e., not inherent.

5. b.

Response: Hand wringing is an expression of a patient's psychic pain. The other answers reflect psychomotor and motor states.

Chapter 5: Laboratory Evaluations and Psychological Testing

1. c.

Response: CNS presentation of medical disease may generate from most organ systems and many pathophysiological mechanisms.

2. a.

Response: Clinical judgment regards appropriate medical rule-ins and rule-outs. Cost/benefit regards the likelihood that test results will alter treatment and how vital this information will be in deciding the treatment course in the context of test costs. Standards of practice in the community are measured as insurance carriers cost-analyze and compare your patterns with those of your local peers and in medicolegal situations. However, in all cases do what you believe is best for the patient, and document your reasoning.

3. b.

Response: The chances of medical explanation for a new onset psychiatric syndrome in an elderly person increase with later age of onset.

4. d.

Response: Therapeutic range for valproate blood levels has been routinely used in clinical management of bipolar disorder

5. d.

Response: The Food and Drug Administration has allowed the release on use of clozapine only with appropriate white blood cell (WBC) and absolute neutrophil count (ANC) being checked once a week for 6 months, then every 2 weeks thereafter. The frequency of effect on WBC and ANC was significant and could be lethal. However, it was found that routine monitoring allowed early intervention by discontinuation of the drug to prevent a severe outcome.

Chapter 6: Diagnostic Impression, Formulation, and Plan

1. d.

Response: Assessment is followed by your plan, describing what other information or tests you need to obtain as well as the therapeutic intervention you plan to do.

2. b.

Response: How you think through analysis of clinical data is what your teachers can help you with as you learn the field. This is important to document to demonstrate your thinking.

3. a.

Response: Different domains include Axis I: Clinical Disorders, other conditions that may be focus of clinical attention; Axis II: Personality Disorders, Mental Retardation; Axis III: General Medical Conditions; Axis IV: Psychosocial and Environmental Problems; and Axis V: Global Assessment of Functioning

4. c.

Response: DSM -IV-TR by convention includes Personality Disorders and Mental Retardation on Axis II.

5. a.

Response: Because cognitive and secondary psychiatric disorders present as a psychiatric syndrome, they are defined as Axis I disorders.

Part III: Psychopathology: Disorders and Clinical Presentations

Chapter 7: Psychiatric Emergencies and Urgent Care Issues

1. a.

Response: Self-destructive acts, although less acutely lethal, are symptomatic of internal distress of the patient and hence require inclusion in assessment of a patient's diagnosis and appropriate treatment plan. Either by mistake of by progressive escalation, these sub-lethal behaviors may elevate into lethality.

2. a.

Response: This is a finding from epidemiological studies of suicide attempts versus completed suicides.

3. d.

Response: The combination of severe Axis I pathology in the context of impulsivity present in Personality Disorder may escalate the risk of suicide over those with Personality Disorder alone.

4. c.

Response: This is a finding from analysis of epidemiological cohort studies.

5. d.

Response: This is a finding from epidemiological studies of completed suicides.

Chapter 8: Cognitive and Secondary ("Organic") Mental Disorders

1. c.

Response: "Organic" versus "functional" was a prevalent clinical distinction a couple decades ago. Organic psychiatric syndromes referred to traditional medical etiology, and functional without such known medical etiology. The term organic still persists in clinical circles and still serves as a useful description.

2. a.

Response: Cognitive domain includes mental functions of attention, consciousness, language, speech, memory, and visuospatial skills.

3. c.

Response: Other choices do not reflect known causes of traditional medical explanation of psychiatric symptoms. Low levels of serotonin are associated with Major Depressive Episode, but although a biological explanation of symptoms, "secondary" connotes arising from specific medical etiologies.

4. d.

Response: An important side effect of theophylline is an anxiogenic effect.

5. c.

Response: Glucocorticoids are known to have a risk of causing manic psychotic depressive or cognitive symptoms.

Chapter 9: Mood Disorders

1. b.

Response: If the average lifetime risk of having a Major Depressive Episode is about 17% and that of bipolar disorder is about 1.6%, then the risk of your patient with a Major Depressive Episode of having a bipolar depression is about 1:10, or 10%.

2. a.

Response: Patients with Bipolar I Disorder (highs have a history of full mania) and Bipolar II Disorder depressed phase with a history of moderate severe hypomania need a mood stabilizer along with antidepressant in order to prevent induction of hypomania or mania. Bipolar II depressed patients with only mild hypomania histories may not need a mood stabilizer with the antidepressant; however, this practice still remains controversial.

3. a.

Response: Anhedonia or depressed mood is required to be present to make a diagnosis of Major Depressive Episode.

4. a.

Response: DSM recognizes mixed episodes as possible in Bipolar I Disorder but not the others. There is currently clinical controversy whether there should be "mixed episodes" in Bipolar II disorder

5. d.

Response: Ruminations are not a psychotic feature of a mood disorder. However, delusions, hallucinations, and disorder of thought forms are considered psychotic.

Chapter 10: Psychotic Disorders

1. d.

Response: Three manifestations of psychosis are hallucinations, delusions, and disorder of thought process or form.

2. c.

Response: None of the other diagnoses have psychotic symptoms as a feature.

3. d.

Response: Definition of term.

4. b.

Response: Negative symptoms are poorly responsive to current treatments compared with positive symptoms.

5. b.

Response: MICA: mental illness chemical abuse. The combined approach of dealing with both the psychiatric and substance abuse diagnoses simultaneously has a better outcome than either approach alone when patients suffer from both problems.

Chapter 11: Anxiety Disorders

1. b.

Response: The amygdala has been noted to coordinate neurobiological responses in these disorders

2. a.

Response: Chest pain can be from chest muscle tension associated with anxiety.

3. c.

Response: Dilation of blood vessels in the face associated with anxiety.

4. b.

Response: His symptoms go beyond that of an adjustment disorder, yet are an anxiety disorder.

5. d.

Response: The panic attack may occur spontaneously away from home, but thereafter being away from home is associated with panic; hence, the fear of leaving home.

Chapter 12: Substance Use Disorders

1. d.

Response: Fact.

2. c.

Response: Definition. Intoxication by different substance have different characteristic behavioral states.

3. d.

Response: Absence of previous symptoms, brief history, association with new acquaintances, the syndrome presentation, associated with stimulant intoxication and positive urine drug screen together make the diagnosis.

4. c.

Response: She has purely physiological dependence, not psychological dependence, on phenobarbital.

5. a.

Response: Acamprosate reduces the physiology associated with the experience of craving alcohol through antagonizing glutamate.

Chapter 13: Personality Traits and Disorders

1. d.

Response: Enduring pattern of these characteristics tend to be lifelong.

2. b.

Response: DSM convention.

3. d.

Response: Major Depression may so shake the person's confidence and self-esteem that the experience state of depression temporarily increases the need for reassurance and support, and the patient appears excessively dependent (if you did not know the baseline behavior). This excessive need for reassurance, support, and other dependent features disappears when the episode of Major Depression is in remission.

4. c.

Response: This is an enduring deviation from the norm, with consequent impairments interpersonally and in other role functioning.

5. c.

Response: DSM conventions of this cluster of personality disorder, which has significant anxiety and fear in common.

Chapter 14: Other Psychopathological Categories

1. c.

Response: Anxiety directly affects parasympathetic outputs to the intestinal tract, contributing to the altered motility of irritable bowel syndrome, thus being a paradigmatic example of psychological factors affecting physical condition.

2. a.

Response: Anxiety directly affects bronchospasm, presumably mediated by parasympathetic outputs.

3. d.

Response: Medically unexplained symptoms often become "explained" later in the illness course as the etiology more definitively declares itself.

4. c.

Response: Panic attacks in panic disorder often manifest with chest discomfort, palpitations, diaphoresis, and nausea, symptoms that are also highly suggestive of cardiac ischemia, often leading to cardiologist consultation.

5. a.

Response: The major depression needs treatment, but one must not assume that concomitant physical symptoms are necessarily due to the depression and must work them up appropriately as well.

Part IV: Psychiatric Treatments

Chapter 15: Psychotherapies

1. c.

Response: Empathy by definition involves putting oneself in the place of another emotionally; it is thus among the most useful and beneficial tools used in the physician-patient relationship.

2. d.

Response: Patients learn how to respond to painful affects by identifying with the role modeling of a physician with whom they have a positive alliance.

3. b.

Response: The statement by the physician informed the patient what to do in certain circumstances, a form of patient education.

4. a.

Response: While in some ways an unsatisfactory term that demeans the skills involved, the term "bedside manner" has long been used to describe the sum total of physicians' interpersonal and communication skills with patients.

5. c.

Response: Exploration of issues surrounding her sexual abuse must wait until resolution of her psychotic depression, a state in which adding to her emotional distress is contraindicated.

Chapter 16: Pharmacotherapy

1. d.

Response: SNRIs such as venlafaxine likely have greater efficacy than SSRIs or non-antidepressant agents in severe major depression with melancholia.

2. b.

Response: "Pharmacogenetics" refers to genetic influences on pharmaco-kinetics or on response to the drug's mechanism of action, which might explain how family history of drug response affects drug response in this patient.

3. b.

Response: Many psychiatric disorders affect motivation, either directly (as in depression) or due to impaired insight into the illness and the need for treatment. The other factors are also relevant, but not necessarily more so for psychiatric patients compared with those with other types of diseases.

4. b.

Response: "Recurrence" by definition is a new episode that occurs after a period of full remission from a prior episode.

5. b.

Response: "Relapse" by definition is a worsening of symptoms during a given episode, i.e., before having reached a period of full remission/recovery.

Chapter 17: Other Somatic Therapies

1. b.

Response: Electroconvulsive therapy works as a safe, reproducible means of inducing a seizure. It is the seizure that is therapeutic, not the electricity itself.

2. a.

Response: Electroconvulsive therapy, like antidepressants, produces down-regulation of beta-adrenergic receptors, probably as a response to stimulation of monoamine release, including norepinephrine.

3. b.

Response: Inflation of the cuff above systolic pressure prevents arterial circulation to that limb; thus, the neuromuscular blockade produced by succinylcholine does not occur, and the motor manifestations of the seizure can be observed in that limb.

4. c.

Response: Tricyclic antidepressants plus lithium augmentation have been shown specifically to prevent recurrence of depression following acute treatment with electroconvulsive therapy.

5. b.

Response: "Neuromodulation" is the term used to describe altered neuronal function via a variety of means, including the use of currents as described.

Part V: Treatment Settings and Subspecialties

Chapter 18: Treatment Settings, Systems, and Other Clinical Issues

1. b.

Response: "Short-term" refers specifically to length of stay. Patient mix, staffing, and other factors may be altered, but the primary criterion for admission to such units is driven by those patients likely to benefit from a short length of stay.

2. c.

Response: On average, day treatment programs are more likely to treat patients for extended periods of time, whereas partial hospital programs are likely to be shorter-term treatments.

3. d.

Response: The consultant is, by definition, consulting with the referring provider; the latter is responsible for direct care to the patient.

4. c.

Response: Psychiatrists are physicians who have undergone specialty training consisting of (at least) 4 years of residency training.

Chapter 19: Psychiatric Subspecialties

1. b.

Response: Whereas the other subspecialties have evolved in light of specialized knowledge and skills in relatively recent years, child and adolescent psychiatry has been recognized for decades as requiring more unique skills.

2. a.

Response: MICA means "mentally ill chemical abusers," i.e., patients with comorbid addictions and other mental illnesses.

Glossary of Frequently Used Psychiatric Terms

This select list of terms was chosen to help you understand more quickly the conversations among clinicians that may be occurring on the wards. Although this list is not exhaustive, it is intended to assist in jargon mastery.

Term	Basic Definition
Alexithymia	Difficulty in describing or recognizing one's own emotions; a common problem in somatoform, addictive, acute stress, and post-traumatic stress disorders
Biofeedback	A method of allowing the patient to learn control over usually imperceptible physiological processes by the use of instrumentation to provide the feedback about one's physiological process (such as blood pressure, muscle tension, brainwave types, etc.)
Catharsis	Having an appropriate and therapeutic release (emotional reaction) in talking out conscious, or becoming aware of unconscious, material
Cognitive	Has two distinct usages: (1) mental process of reasoning, as in cognitive psychology and cognitive therapy; (2) intellectual functions including attention, memory, language, praxis, and others, as in cognitive testing and cognitive disorders
Commitment	Legal process of admitting a mentally ill patient to a psychiatric facility; process may be voluntary but more often refers to involuntary admission

Countertransference	The clinician's unconscious emotional reaction to the patient, determined by the clinician's own needs and perceptions
Day hospital	Some services similar to those of inpatient hospitalization but patients go home at night; are usually several days per week; a level of acuity between regular outpatient care and inpatient hospitalization; also called *partial hospitalization*
Functional (symptom or disorder)	Term for changes in the operation of an organ system, in which no identifiable structural disturbance can be found
Logorrhea	Talking that is excessive and uncontrolled
Milieu therapy	An essential part of inpatient psychiatric treatment in which everyday events and interactions are therapeutically designed for the purpose of enhancing social skills, building confidence, and improving stability
Mind	Integration of the functions of the brain, resulting in the ability to perceive, think, feel, imagine, remember, have will, and process information in an intelligent manner
Nervous breakdown	A nonmedical term (more often used by patients) that refers to any acute mental illness or condition that interferes with normal function, action, or thought
Neuroleptic	An older term for an antipsychotic drug
Object relations	Emotional attachments for people or things and how the person's relationship with them is incorporated into self
Organic	Characterized by a detectable or observable change in tissues or organs in the body; sometimes used as antonym of "functional"
Perception	The mind's interpretation of its organization of emotional, intellectual, or sensory data
Psychomotor	Physical activity associated with mental processes
Psychosomatic	Disorder that has a physiological component but thought to originate in or made worse by the person's emotional state; sometimes called *psychophysiological*

Term	Basic Definition (continued)
Psychotherapy	Verbal therapy between a clinician and a patient (individual) or many patients (group); many different types of psychotherapy, based on the theories behind the therapeutic interventions
Somatic therapy	Biological treatment of psychiatric disorders, such as by medications, electroconvulsive therapy, and light therapy; often contrasted to psychotherapy
Transference	Unconscious assignment (transfer) of negative or positive feelings that were originally associated with significant figures from the past (often parents or siblings) onto a current person in a person's life; term commonly refers to feelings transferred onto the clinician by the patient

ABBREVIATIONS

This select list of abbreviations was chosen to help you understand more quickly the conversations among clinicians that may be occurring on the wards. Although this list is not exhaustive, it is intended to assist in jargon mastery.

Abbreviation	Complete Term
5-HT	5-hydroxytryptamine (serotonin)
5-HT2	5-hydroxytryptamine-2 (serotonin-2) (postsynaptic)
AA	Alcoholics Anonymous
ABPN	American Board of Psychiatry and Neurology
ACE	Angiotensin-converting enzyme
ACTH	Adrenocorticotropic hormone
ADHD	Attention-deficit/hyperactivity disorder
AMA	Against medical advice
AMI	Amitriptyline
ANC	Absolute neutrophil count
AV	Atrioventricular
BDNF	Brain-derived neurotropic factor
BPD	Borderline personality disorder
BUN	Blood urea nitrogen
CAD	Coronary artery disease
c-AMP	Cyclic adenosine monophosphate
CBC	Complete blood count
CBT	Cognitive behavioral therapy
CC	Chief complaint
CD	Chemical dependency
C-L	Consultation-Liaison
CMI	Clomipramine
CNS	Central nervous system

Abbreviation	Complete Term (continued)
CPK	Creatine phosphokinase
CPZ	Chlorpromazine
CREB	Cyclic AMP response element binding
CRF or CRH	Corticotropin-releasing factor (or corticotropin-releasing hormone)
CT	Computed tomography
CXR	Chest x-ray
CYP	Cytochrome P-450
DBS	Deep-brain stimulation
DBT	Dialectical behavioral therapy
DMC	Decision-making capacity
DMI	Desipramine
DNRI	Dopamine norepinephrine reuptake inhibitor
DSM	*Diagnostic and Statistical Manual of Mental Disorders* (current edition = DSM-IV-TR; see "A Note about DSM Editions" in the Preface)
DTP	Day treatment program
Dx or dx	Diagnosis
ECG	Electrocardiogram
ECT	Electroconvulsive therapy
EEG	Electroencephalogram
EPS	Extrapyramidal side effects
FDA	U.S. Food and Drug Administration
FEF	Frontal executive function
GABA	Gamma-amino butyric acid
GAD	Generalized anxiety disorder
GAF	Global assessment of functioning
GI	Gastrointestinal
GFR	Glomerular filtration rate
HCP	Health-care proxy
HDL	High-density lipoprotein
HEENT	Head, eyes, ears, nose, throat
HIV	Human immunodeficiency virus
HMO	Health maintenance organization
HPI	History of present illness
Hx	History
ICM	Intensive case manager
IM	Intramuscular
IMI	Imipramine
IPT	Interpersonal psychotherapy

IQ	Intelligence quotient
IR	Immediate release
IV	Intravenous
LBBB	Left bundle-branch block
LFT	Liver function test value
LOC	Level of consciousness
LOS	Length of stay
LP	Lumbar puncture
LSD	Lysergic acid diethylamide
MAO-A	Monoamine oxidase-A
MAO-B	Monoamine oxidase-B
MAOI	Monoamine oxidase inhibitor
MDD	Major depressive disorder
MDE	Major depressive episode
MI	Myocardial infarction
MICA	Mentally ill chemical abuser
MMSE	Mini-Mental Status Examination
MR	Mental retardation
MRDD	Mental Retardation or Developmental Disabilities
MRI	Magnetic resonance imaging
MSE	Mental status examination
MUS	Medically unexplained symptoms
NaSSA	Norepinephrine and specific serotonin antidepressant
NGF	Nerve growth factor
NMDA	N-methyl-D-aspartate
NMS	Neuroleptic malignant syndrome
NOS	Not otherwise specified
NSAID	Nonsteroidal anti-inflammatory drug
NTP	Nortriptyline
OCD	Obsessive-compulsive disorder
PCP	Primary care physician *or* phencyclidine
PE	Physical examination
PET	Positron emission tomography
PHP	Partial hospital program
PO	By mouth *(per os)*
PRN	As necessary *(pro re nata)*
PSM	Psychosomatic medicine
PTSD	Post-traumatic stress disorder
REM	Rapid eye movement
RIMA	Reversible inhibitor of monoamine oxidase-A

Term	Complete Term (continued)
ROS	Review of systems
RPR	Rapid plasma reagin
rTMS	Repetitive transcranial magnetic stimulation
SAD	Seasonal affective disorder
SI	Suicidal ideation
SIB	Self-injurious behavior
SNRI	Serotonin norepinephrine reuptake inhibitor
SPECT	Single photon emission computed tomography
SPMI	Severely and persistently mentally ill
SR	Sustained release
SSRI	Selective serotonin reuptake inhibitor
TCA	Tricyclic antidepressant
TD	Tardive dyskinesia
TSH	Thyroid-stimulating hormone
Tx *or* tx	Treatment
VNS	Vagus nerve stimulation
WBC	White blood cell
XR	Extended-release

APPENDIX

D

KEY CONTACTS AND NOTES

Physician Contacts

NAME	CONTACT
Dr	Home phone: Mobile phone: Pager: Other:
Dr	Home phone: Mobile phone: Pager: Other:
Dr	Home phone: Mobile phone: Pager: Other:
Dr	Home phone: Mobile phone: Pager: Other:
Dr	Home phone: Mobile phone: Pager: Other:
Dr	Home phone: Mobile phone: Pager: Other:

Community Resources and Phone Numbers

NAME/PROGRAM	PHONE NUMBERS
Sexual and Physical Abuse	
Substance Abuse	
Communicable Diseases (HIV, Hepatitis, Others)	
Homeless Shelters	
Child/Adolescent Hotlines	

Community Resources and Phone Numbers

NAME/PROGRAM   PHONE NUMBERS

Suicide Hotlines

Hospitals (General,
Veterans, Psychiatric)

Medicare

Medicaid

Other

Facility Phone Numbers

NAME/PROGRAM	PHONE NUMBERS
Main	Phone:
	Fax:
	Phone:
	Fax:
Laboratory	Phone:
	Fax:
	Phone:
	Fax:
Radiology	Phone:
	Fax:
	Phone:
	Fax:
Physical therapy	Phone:
	Fax:
	Phone:
	Fax:
ECG/EEG	Phone:
	Fax:
	Phone:
	Fax:
Outpatient Scheduling	Phone:
	Fax:
	Phone:
	Fax:
Emergency	Phone:
	Fax:
	Phone:
	Fax:
Operating Suite	Phone:
	Fax:
	Phone:
	Fax:

Facility Phone Numbers

NAME/PROGRAM	PHONE NUMBERS
Admissions	Phone:
	Fax:
	Phone:
	Fax:
Billing	Phone:
	Fax:
	Phone:
	Fax:
Medical Records	Phone:
	Fax:
	Phone:
	Fax:
Medical Staff Office	Phone:
	Fax:
	Phone:
	Fax:
Other important numbers	Phone:
	Fax:
	Phone:
	Fax:
Other important numbers	Phone:
	Fax:
	Phone:
	Fax:
Other important numbers	Phone:
	Fax:
	Phone:
	Fax
Other important numbers	Phone:
	Fax:
	Phone:
	Fax

Formulary Notes Specific to Your Facility

Other Important Information

Index

Psychostimulant, 251
Psychosurgery
  ablative, 276–277
  deep brain stimulation, 277
  neuromodulation, 277
Psychotherapist, 299
Psychotherapy, 336
  behavioral and cognitive,
    221–222, 222b
  brief psychodynamic, 220–221
  for children, 314
  doctor-patient relationship in,
    212–214
  features of, 186
  formal versus informal, 214
  group, 223–225
  mentor tips for, 227
  overview of, 211
  supportive-expressive continuum
    expressive, 216, 218, 219t
    overview of, 214–215
    supportive, 215–216, 217t
  techniques for, 187
Psychotic disorder
  Brief Psychotic Disorder, 143
  delusional disorder, 144–146
  mentor tips for, 147–148
  schizoaffective disorder, 143–144
  schizophrenia, 139–142
  schizophreniform disorder, 142–143
  shared, 147
  symptoms of, 139
Publicly-funded long-term unit, 289
Pyromania, 203

R

Reaction formation, 16t
Reasoning, emotional, 19t
Repetitive transcranial magnetic
  stimulation (rTMS), 278
Repression, 16t
Review of systems (ROS), 35–39
Ropinirole (Requip), 262
Ruminative thinking
  as a symptom, 74t

S

Schizoaffective disorder
  overview of, 143–144
  spectrum of, 145f
Schizoid personality disorder, 179, 188
Schizophrenia, 139–142, 188
  in children, 313–314
Schizophreniform disorder
  brief psychotic disorder, comparing
    to, 144t
  overview of, 142–143
Schizotypal personality
  disorder, 179–180
Seasonal affective disorder (SAD)
  light therapy for, 278–280
  prevention of, 281
Secondary mental disorder
  overview and etiology of, 97–99
  types of, 103
Second-generation antipsychotic
  overview of, 237
Selective abstraction, 19t
Selective serotonin reuptake inhibitor
  (SSRI), 247–248
Selective Serotonin Reuptake Inhibitor
  (SSRI) Discontinuation Syndrome,
  94, 96–97
Self-destructive acts, 82t–83t
Serotonin-norepinephrine reuptake
  inhibitor (SNRI), 245, 247
Serotonin Syndrome
  Neuroleptic Malignant Syndrome
    (NMS), comparing to, 95t–96t
  as psychiatric emergency, 93–94
Severely and persistently mentally ill
  (SPMI), 300–301
Sexual dysfunction, 202–203
Shared psychotic disorder, 147
Short-term unit, 286–287
Should statement, 19t
Side effects, pharmacotherapy, 230–231
Sleep architecture, 13
Sleep disorder
  classification of, 205
  overview of, 204
Sleep terror, 206

359

Trauma, psychological, 89–90
Trazodone, 248
Treatment
 for children, 314–315
 issues affecting, 7
 mentor tips for, 9, 9–10, 307–308
 multidisciplinary roles/teams for
  activity therapist, 299
  nurse, 297–298
  overview of, 295
  paraprofessional, 299
  psychiatrist, 296
  psychotherapist, 299
  social worker, 298–299
 phenomenology and, 5–6
 in psychiatry, 6
 selection of, 7, 9–10
 settings for
  inpatient psychiatric unit, 286–289
  outpatient programs, 290–291
  partial hospital and day treatment
   programs, 289–290
  psychiatric emergency room, 294–295
 systems of care for, 300

 types of, 287–288
 See also Psychotherapy
Trichotillomania, 204
Tricyclic antidepressant (TCA),
 244–245, 246t–247t
Tyramine-induced hypertensive
 crisis, 97

U
Unconsciousness, 14
Undifferentiated Somatoform
 Disorder, 196

V
Vagus nerve stimulation (VNS), 277
Valproic acid, 257
Violence
 management of, 88–89
 overview and risk factors for, 87–88
Visuospatial skills, 55

W
Work week adjustment, 278, 280f